pilates *for the* outdoor athlete

LAURI ANN STRICKER

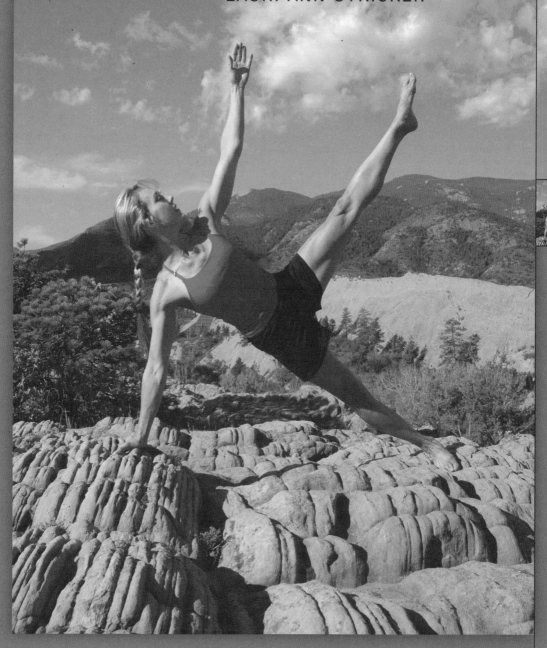

FULCRUM PUBLISHING
WWW.FULCRUMBOOKS.COM

PHOTO CREDITS:
Page v: Courtesy of Eric McCallister
Pages 1, 6–7, 9, 10: Courtesy of the Pilates
    Method Alliance®
Page 51: Courtesy of Katie Cahill Volpe
Pages 61, 91, 97, 103: © Randy Levensaler
Pages 71, 81: Courtesy of Rachel Linger
Page 115: Courtesy of Raoul Rossiter

    This book is written as a source of infor-
mation only. The information contained in
this book should by no means be considered a
substitute for the advice of a qualified medical
professional, who should always be consulted
before beginning any new exercise or other
health program. The author and the publisher
expressly disclaim responsibility for any
adverse effects arising from the use or applica-
tion of the information contained herein.

Library of Congress
Cataloging-in-Publication Data

Stricker, Lauri Ann.
  Pilates for the outdoor athlete / by Lauri
Ann Stricker.
      p. cm.
  Includes bibliographical references and
index.
  ISBN-13: 978-1-55591-591-9
  ISBN-10: 1-55591-591-4
  1. Pilates method. 2. Physical fitness. 3.
Exercise. I. Title.
  RA781.4.S77 2006
  613.7'1--dc22

2006018659

Printed in China by P. Chan & Edward, Inc.

0 9 8 7 6 5 4 3 2 1

Design: Ann W. Douden
Editorial: Faith Marcovecchio, Jill Amack,
Haley Berry

Fulcrum Publishing
4690 Table Mountain Drive, Suite 100
Golden, Colorado 80403
800-992-2908 • 303-277-1623
www.fulcrumbooks.com

Contents

Your Toolbox

More Tools

Foreword

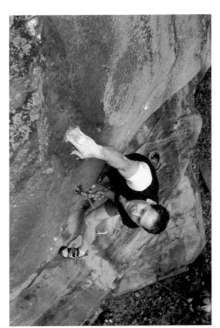

Eric Hörst on the First Ascent on the Logotherapy (5.13a/b), New River Gorge.

As an outdoor athlete of thirty years, I've come to realize that no matter what activity I choose to engage in, the essence of the experience is the movement and the potential for self-discovery. Whether I'm running a rocky trail, skiing fresh powder, or ascending a sheer cliff, it's the kinesthetic experience of moving through nature that nurtures a true sense of pleasure in my soul. Along the way the experience is further enhanced by opportunities to stretch my physical abilities, challenge fears, and test technical skills. In a most elemental sense, I feel that the act of recreating outdoors allows me to constantly re-create myself.

Pilates offers a different pathway to experiencing the joy of movement and self-discovery. For the outdoor athlete, Pilates also offers an effective method of cross-training that can enhance your performance and quality of experience. Given a commitment to train with Pilates a few days per week, you will benefit from improved flexibility, kinesthetic awareness, and breath control. Pilates will also improve strength and stability of your core—the workhorse group of torso muscles that are the foundation for all physical movement. Regular Pilates training can help correct muscle imbalances that inevitably develop in all athletes, and it can go a long way to help prevent many injuries. Finally, Pilates will foster the ability to relax and return to center in stressful situations, and it therefore holds the potential to improve performance in all you do inside or outside.

If these benefits sound alluring, then you are holding the book to make them your reality. Lauri Stricker's *Pilates for the Outdoor Athlete* provides clear, expert instruction that you can put to work, beginning today. Make no mistake—this book is not a rehashing of the basic Pilates instruction found in other books or infomercial products designed for flabby business-men and desperate housewives. As the title states, *Pilates for the Outdoor Athlete* is a text crafted by an accomplished athlete for other athletes looking to elevate their game.

I am fortunate to have known Lauri for a few years now, and I trust that you too will soon share in this fortune by reading this book. Page after page shines with the passion Lauri possesses for this subject, and her genuine desire to help others toward self-actualization is similarly obvious. Lauri is a tremendous spirit, and her energy and knowledge will enrich everyone who reads *Pilates for the Outdoor Athlete*.

I wish you abundant energy, good health, and a life full of transcending experience, joy, and wonder.

—Eric J. Hörst, rock climber, performance coach,
 and author of *Training for Climbing* and *Mental Wings*
 www.EricHorst.com

Acknowledgments

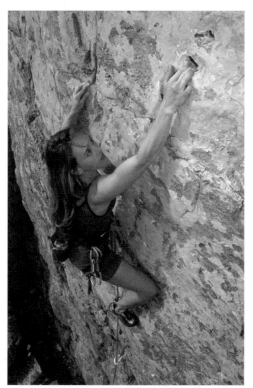

Writing a book is a lot like climbing a steep, powerful short pitch—relentlessly challenging, yet the end is always in sight. And like climbing, the journey is less formidable with someone to hold your rope and offer encouragement as you find your way.

I would like to thank Stewart Green for taking the photo of me that appeared in *Training for Climbing*, a photo that led me to meet Eric J. Hörst, who suggested that I write this book and then helped me find my publisher. Thank you, Eric, for helping me to "spread my mental wings." Thank you, Stewart, for providing me with so many wonderful photos for the book. Thank you, Sam Scinta, Tammy Deranleau, Faith Marcovecchio, and Ann Douden at Fulcrum Publishing, for believing in this project and for all of your hard work.

A big thanks to the people who plowed through the first really awful draft of this book and offered me their insightful feedback. These people include my husband, Kevin, Julie Williamson, Mary Claire (MC) Cahill, and Eric J. Hörst. Thank you, Milena Kirkova, for your beautiful illustrations.

Thank you, Richard Rossiter, my first Pilates mentor, for encouraging and inspiring me to teach and for providing me with a solid foundation of the work. Thank you, Bonnie Grebe, for sharing with me your pearls of wisdom. Thank you to all of my clients for giving me the opportunity to be your coach and to grow as a teacher. Thank you for asking me each week, "How's the book coming along?" Knowing that I was accountable to all of you helped me stay on track, especially when I really wanted to go climbing.

Thank you, Mom and Dad, for your unconditional love, guidance, and for teaching me through example how to live my dreams. Finally, I want to thank my husband, Kevin, for being the best belayer in climbing and life. Thank you, sweetheart, for your love and support, not only in writing this book, but also in creating the life I love.

Introduction

Live in the sunshine,
swim the sea,
drink the wild air …
—RALPH WALDO EMERSON

The Outdoor Athlete

To feel warm sunshine on your face and a cool breeze against your skin, nothing compares to doing what you love in the great outdoors. As outdoor athletes, we train in the gym out of necessity, but we thrive beneath the great blue sky. Our adventures lead us racing out the door after work for trail runs, peddling our bikes on dewy mornings, and waking up before dawn seeking freshly powdered slopes. We spend weekends and vacations pushing our bodies in the heat and cold, rain or shine. Seasons are marked by the number of days spent in the mountains, deserts, and on the rivers. Adventures are reminisced through the friendships we've made. We seek adventure in order to play, test our limits, and to leave different from when we arrived. It's here, under the great blue sky, that we learn our greatest lessons, gain our best insight, and meet our closest friends, partners, and mentors.

Many athletes think that sports are all they need to stay fit and healthy. Although sports build strength and increase cardiovascular endurance, they also create muscle imbalances that can lead to injury. The harder you play, the more important cross-training becomes to keep your muscles balanced, flexible, and resilient. And because outdoor sports mean adventure, mental training is equally important. Pilates cross-training works the body and mind in harmony. When equally strong, the spirit is free to soar. Staying fit and injury free are key to enjoying sports and life for many years to come. This book provides you with the tools for effective Pilates cross-training based on your needs. By practicing a program that is designed especially for your sport, you'll play harder and longer for many years to come.

As outdoor athletes, adventure often calls us to places where we don't have access to a gym and we need to warm up quickly without wasting energy in the process. *Pilates for the Outdoor Athlete* is adaptable to your lifestyle and training schedule so you may achieve your highest aspirations.

Pilates—The Ultimate Cross-Training

Over the past 60 years, the Pilates Method of body conditioning has been proven to be a superior form of cross-training for all athletes. Football players, golfers, tennis players, and triathletes practice Pilates to stay injury free and to perform their best. Until recently, Pilates was only available to those with loads of cash to spend on lessons at exclusive studios. Now virtually every gym across the nation offers Pilates classes, and it can also be easily practiced in your home. This book will empower you to do Pilates safely and effectively on your own time, in your own space, practicing cross-training routines designed specifically for your sport.

Pilates and outdoor sports both require the following skills: concentration and awareness, control, core centering, precision, proper body alignment, natural flowing movement, efficient breathing, and a body-mind connection. As an outdoor athlete pursuing your passion and performing your best, it is critical to stay injury free. Pilates helps you do this by improving muscle balance, flexibility, core strength, alignment, and overall movement skills.

Pilates is a superior form of cross-training because it:

- Improves breathing, circulation, and muscular endurance

- Develops uniformly strong and flexible muscles, thereby reducing muscle imbalance and the likelihood of injury

- Improves efficiency of movement through improved posture and movement skills

- Improves balance by improving core strength, awareness, and movement skills

- Strengthens the mind-body connection, thereby improving mental focus, awareness, and concentration

Once you start doing Pilates, you'll notice yourself incorporating Pilates principles into your sports and daily life. You'll find yourself slouching less, engaging your core more, standing taller, and moving with greater ease. Pilates helps outdoor athletes accomplish three things:

1 Prevent Sport-Specific Injuries

What do climbing, cycling, running, skiing, kayaking, and hiking all have in common? They all perpetuate muscle imbalances through repetitive movement. Have you ever tried to guess what sport someone does based on his predominant muscle mass? Cyclists are easy to spot—quads of steel. So are climbers—forearms the size of bricks and lats like boat oars. As athletes, we tend to overdevelop some muscles and underdevelop others. The outcome: lack of flexibility, poor biomechanics, and joint instability that leads to common injuries such as tendonitis, bursitis, and dislocations. Injuries can mean weeks and months away from what you love to do. Worse yet, once you've developed an injury such as tendonitis, your risk of it becoming chronic looms large. Once you've had an injury to one side of the body, the other side will pick up the slack. This can create imbalances that last long after the injury has healed. Pilates focuses on developing uniform muscles top to bottom, front to back, and left to right, enabling athletes to perform better and avoid injury. Whether you've sustained an injury or managed to fly beneath the radar, Pilates can help you maintain and/or regain the integrity of your body.

2 Improve Performance

Pilates is essentially movement training. All of your movements, whether they're to run and ski or lift heavy boxes and groceries, are improved by doing Pilates. Pilates improves your performance by improving your balance, coordination, posture, breathing, and movement skills. Pilates exercises are designed to work your body and mind in harmony. Therefore, you'll also improve your confidence, mental focus, and clarity. Whether you cycle, ski, climb, kayak, or run, you will develop an efficiency and ease not previously known. Whether your goal is to compete in a triathlon, climb El Capitan, or sea kayak British Columbia's Inside Passage and Vancouver Island Coast, Pilates is your secret weapon for achieving your goals. When you improve the quality of your movements, you become graceful and energy efficient, and improve your endurance. Pilates will improve your posture, alignment, and skills. By doing Pilates, you'll improve your form.

3 Maintain Longevity

Maintaining longevity means moving freely and maintaining flexibility and strength in both the body and mind. One of my lifetime goals is to climb, hike, and snowboard until I'm a granny. Sharing the summit of a Colorado Fourteener with fellow hikers in their 70s makes an impression. By taking better care of your body, mind, and spirit today, you'll improve the quality of your later years.

Pilates is the perfect cross-training program to complement a healthy diet and lifestyle. Balancing your muscles, improving flexibility, and boosting core strength go a long way toward improving longevity. Over the years your goals and sports may change, but your desire to be active in the outdoors will remain. Not only will Pilates improve your longevity as an athlete, it will improve the quality of your life.

15 Minutes a Day

Pilates for the Outdoor Athlete empowers you to cross-train anywhere, anytime. All you need are a flat piece of ground, a mat, a stretch band, and 15 minutes of dedicated time.

This book focuses on seven categories of outdoor athletes: climbers; road cyclists and mountain bikers; hikers, snowshoers, and backpackers; paddlers; road and trail runners; skiers and snowboarders; and multisport athletes. Each of seven sport-specific chapters identifies the benefits of practicing Pilates, common overuse injuries, muscle imbalances, and key muscle groups needing strengthening and stretching to bring the body into balance. The routines are tailored to the athlete, because what an avid climber needs may be dramatically different from what a cyclist or skier needs. The prescriptions are designed with the lifestyle of the outdoor athlete in mind. Utilizing powerful imagery and concise cues, you'll be able to perform high-quality movement and garner results:

- Boost core strength

- Solidify movement patterns and reinforce proper alignment

Introduction

3

- Strengthen antagonist (nonsport-specific) muscles and improve joint integrity

- Improve flexibility, range of motion, and recovery of agonist (sport-specific) muscles

Why Only 15 Minutes?

Just about everyone can find 15 minutes three to five times a week to practice Pilates. The short time commitment encourages you to practice frequently and produces quicker results than longer sessions done less often. Practicing three to five days a week helps reinforce new movement skills and better posture and alignment. In addition, the short format emphasizes quality over quantity. Repetitions are low and focus on working the body uniformly. You want to be mentally focused throughout your entire routine.

By practicing regularly, you'll find yourself developing strength and flexibility faster. The routines will complement and enhance your sports training, making you a stronger, more flexible, and more focused athlete.

Frequently Asked Questions

Who is doing Pilates and getting results? Triathletes, skiers, and climbers are just a few of the outdoor athletes who are practicing Pilates. Once thought to be something only for dancers, Pilates is a well-practiced form of cross-training among professional football and basketball players, golfers, tennis players, and even bull riders.

How is Pilates different from yoga? Pilates is movement training with an emphasis on alignment, breathing, and core conditioning. Pilates practitioners create a scooped-out midsection, which is different from most forms of yoga, in which practitioners often breathe into the belly. In addition, while yoga tends to be meditational in intention, Pilates is an exercise regimen. Both Pilates and yoga share the common goal of balancing the body and training your mind and body as an integrated whole.

How much time is involved, and what's the learning curve? Using the program outlined in this book, you will be on your way to seeing results within the first six weeks of practice. Do the routine for 15 minutes, three to five times per week, and you'll not only move differently, but you'll also look and feel different.

Do I need to take a class? It is not necessary to take a class prior to beginning your Pilates cross-training. However, if you have special needs or want to ensure proper alignment, taking a class can provide great benefit. To find a qualified instructor, I recommend visiting www.pilatesmethodalliance.org.

What's the difference between studio equipment work and mat? Unlike mat work, the apparatus work is more easily adapted to create more or less challenge. This is beneficial for people recovering from injury or without sufficient core strength to do the mat work. Equipment work is also great for athletes who want to expand their practice beyond the mat work. The mat work is perfect if you are reasonably fit and want to the freedom to do the work on your own time and in your own space. All of the mat work outlined in this book is portable, doesn't require a membership, and is available 24/7.

Chapter 1

Joseph Pilates and His Method

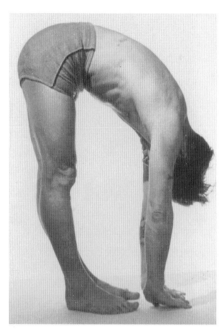

Who's the German Guy?

I cannot tell you how many times I've taught a class in which not a single person knew that Joe Pilates was a real person. It's time to give the guy credit. Not only was Joe a real person, he was a hard-core athlete who skied, swam, boxed, and at one time performed in a circus. A self-proclaimed visionary who knew that he was 50 years ahead of his time, Joe created the Pilates Method of physical and mental conditioning, which is applied by athletes all over the world. Contrary to popular belief, Joe was not a dancer.

Like many visionaries, Joe triumphed over great adversity. The story goes like this: Joe was born in 1880 and grew up in Düsseldorf, Germany, where as a child he suffered from rickets, asthma, and rheumatic fever. Determined to overcome his illnesses, he devised a system to increase his physical vitality and fitness. By the time he was a teenager, not only had he overcome his frailties, he had become so fit that he was asked to pose in his skivvies for anatomical drawings of the human body. Not bad, eh? Overcoming his own battles with sickness as a child created in him a belief in the body's ability to heal—so long as the mind led. He believed that our body should obey our will and not vice versa. His favorite quote is said to have been by Friederich von Schiller: "It is Spirit itself that builds the body."

In 1912 Joe went to England, and when World War I erupted he was incarcerated on the Isle of Man with other German nationals as an enemy alien. While incarcerated, he shared his method of fitness, the mat work, with his fellow compatriots. It was so effective that in 1918, when an epidemic of influenza spread through England killing thousands, not a single person in the camp who trained with Joe became ill. His training system improved not only their immune systems but their mental well-being and sense of personal power as well. While interned Joe also helped bedridden people in the infirmary become fitter and healthier. He removed the box springs from their beds and attached them to the wall behind them. Tying slings to the ends of the springs, Joe enabled people to exercise their arms and legs while lying in a stable position. Imagine a stocky German guy standing over your bed saying, "Okay, you're not dead—start exercising." The results were astonishing: people became stronger and healthier. This was only the beginning. These early ideas led Joe to develop the apparatus presently being used in Pilates studios and physical therapy settings worldwide. Today, Pilates is widely used as rehabilitative exercise for soft-tissue injury and to alleviate back pain caused by injury, faulty

biomechanics, and inadequate core strength.

In 1926 Joe came to the United States and opened a studio in New York City. On the boat over, he met his wife, Clara, who became instrumental in teaching his method. Together they opened a studio in the same building as the New York City Ballet. Dancers studying under the tutelage of Martha Graham and George Balanchine were among his biggest fans. Joe helped them to recover from injury, improve their performance, and increase their longevity as dancers. As a result, the majority of Joe's first- and second-generation teachers are dancers.

Joe's Crew

It is because of the dedication and commitment of Joseph Pilates' wife, Clara, and his original students that the Pilates Method lived on after his death in 1967. The most formidable and influential of Joe's protégés have been Mary Bowen, Ron Fletcher, Eve Gentry, Kathy Grant, Bruce King, Romana Kryzanowska, and Lolita San Miguel. Each one is considered a master or elder teacher who has produced a strong lineage. Each lineage shares the six universally accepted principles, which will be discussed later in this chapter, and is distinct in its techniques, reflecting the personality and experience of the master teacher.

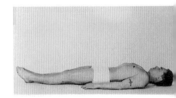

Joe's Book: *Return to Life*

In 1945 Joe wrote *Return to Life through Contrology*. By his definition, "Contrology develops the body uniformly, corrects wrong postures, restores physical vitality, invigorates the mind, and elevates the spirit." *Return to Life* contains 34 mat exercises and is the unequivocal source for Pilates mat exercise information. In his book Joe shares his philosophy regarding fitness, diet, sleep, and lifestyle. He believed that spending time in nature pursuing recreational activities was critical to counteract the effects of too much work and stress. As he expresses the importance of exercise and breathing fresh air, I easily recognize him as a fellow hiker I might nod to some brisk autumn morning.

Pilates for Athletes

Joe created his method with an end in mind: "The attainment and maintenance of a uniformly developed body with a sound mind fully capable of naturally, easily, and satisfactorily performing our many and varied daily tasks with spontaneous zest and pleasure." When asked by his students, as he often was, "Joe, what's this for, why am I doing this exercise?" Joe was known to say, "It'z for zee body." Unlike a typical strength-training workout, Pilates doesn't work legs today and arms tomorrow, for example. It is designed to work your entire body uniformly each session. Pilates requires the participation of all the muscles. As you switch from one movement to the next, you'll build flexibility, strength,

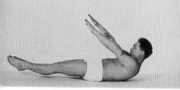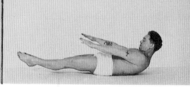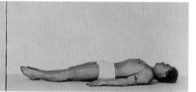

Joe performs the Hundred.

and stamina. Pilates strengthens and stretches all parts of your body, front to back, left to right, and top to bottom. As an athlete, muscle imbalances are common and require targeting our training to areas to achieve uniform development. *Pilates for the Outdoor Athlete* addresses the muscle imbalances created by sports and applies specific exercises to restore integrity to the body.

The Big Six

Pilates is based on six principles that apply to athletics: breathing, centering, concentration, control, fluid motion, and precision. Implementing these six principles to everyday movement such as walking, loading a backpack, or climbing a set of stairs will change the way you look, feel, and move in your body. As you integrate the six principles into your life and sports, you'll be on your way to becoming more fit and energetic in your sports and for the rest of your life.

1 Breathing

Breath is the spirit of our being—it is our life force. As athletes, proper breathing fuels our movements, calms our mind, and reduces fatigue. Yet many of us hold our breath, hyperventilate, breathe shallowly, or have never considered the role of breathing in athletics. Proper breathing is essential to our heart and enables our muscles to work optimally. As athletes, we know the burning sensation brought on by a deficit of oxygen as lactic acid fills our limbs. Like a flowing river moving water to the sea, proper breathing pumps oxygen-rich blood into each muscle, cleaning the bloodstream and improving circulation. In his book, Joe said, "Lazy breathing converts the lungs, figuratively speaking, into a cemetery for the deposition of diseased, dying, and dead germs as well as supplying an ideal haven for the multiplication of other harmful germs." Sounds pretty grim.

Pilates breathing emphasizes inhaling through the nose and exhaling out the mouth. Nose breathing stimulates the parasympathetic nervous system and produces hormones that enhance our physiology. These hormones decrease heart rate and blood pressure and have a calming effect on the body. Conversely, mouth breathing stimulates the sympathetic nervous system, quickening the heart rate and producing hormones associated with flight-or-fight emotions. Next time you are feeling really tense while engaged in your sport, notice your breathing. Inhaling through your nose calms your mind, helps you monitor your heart rate and exertion levels, and causes you to become dehydrated less quickly than mouth breathing.

Joe told his students to exhale forcefully as if they were wringing water out of a dishtowel. He said, "This is the equivalent of an 'internal shower.'" Forceful exhalation taps into the deepest layer of abdominal muscle, the transverse abdominis (TA), creating support for our spines, massaging our vital organs, and helping us to align our bodies more effectively. An effective technique for proper breathing is to imagine your rib cage as an old-fashioned umbrella. As you inhale, the umbrella opens. As you exhale, you close the umbrella, forcing all the air out. Another way to think about this is to narrow the center of your waist like an hourglass. This technique stretches and strengthens the muscles along the spine, freeing you to bend, twist, and rotate more easily.

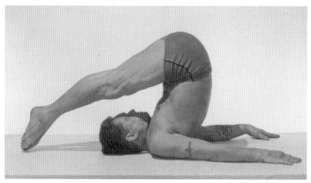

Joe performs the Roll Over.

2 Centering

Core-centered movement supports the low back, increases your power, and improves your posture and alignment. In Pilates every movement is initiated from the "core" or "center": what Joe referred to as the "powerhouse." This area includes the abdominal, lower back, and hip muscles. Maintaining a strong center supports proper alignment and good posture. A strong core is necessary to maintain a stable pelvis to support the lower back as well as to help maintain optimal alignment. As athletes, tapping into your center not only improves alignment, but it makes sports movements easier and less tiring. Your limbs fatigue less

quickly when the back is better supported. The center's integrity affects the entire unit. The strength of your "powerhouse" determines the efficiency, power, and grace of your movements.

3 Concentration

Athletes perform their best when they stay present in the moment. Improving concentration helps tap into the "zone," where the body and mind are synchronized and distractions are distant and pale. A focused athlete is a safer athlete. Pilates brings the mind and body into harmony by engaging them equally, a state Joe called contrology: "Contrology is the complete coordination of body, mind, and spirit." Joseph Pilates knew that what happens in the mind precedes the body. Therefore, Pilates demands that you focus your mind on the activity of your body. Focus on what it is you are trying to accomplish. You can improve your concentration by learning to breathe deeply and visualize the movements you want to create. It's easy to get distracted and start worrying about work or thinking about what you're going to do later. If you find yourself distracted, pick one thing about the exercise that you can really focus on and tune into it completely. The same is true when you run, kayak, or do any other sport: give your attention to it completely. Focus on enjoying the movement, and you'll be more tuned in to your body.

4 Control

Control means creating movements that are intentional, calculated, and, well, controlled. Controlled movements are energy efficient, reduce your risk of injury, and improve your form. Imagine Lance Armstrong cycling out of control. Imagine climber Lynn Hill thrashing up El Capitan out of control. It just doesn't happen. You cannot perform your best if your movements are erratic, sloppy, haphazard, and damaging to your body. Strive to execute all movements with intention, awareness, and control.

5 Fluid Motion

Fluid motion is smooth and effortless movement that minimizes wear and tear on your joints, saves energy, and improves enjoyment. Pilates exercises are to be done with grace and efficiency. Once you understand a movement, the body-mind can take over and you no longer have to think about it, you simply feel it. Fluid motion is easier on your joints.

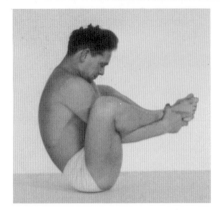

Joe and the Seal.

6 Precision

Precision starts with an awareness of your alignment. By improving your precision, you'll improve your movement biomechanics, minimize energy expenditure, and reduce the risk of injury. Watch an expert skier take the bumps, and you'll see precise turns down the fall line. Observe a talented climber scaling the underside of a cave, and it's as though she's performing a ballet. Exact movement with the right amount of energy requires precision. Pilates demands and cultivates precision. Improving our alignment, core strength, and concentration improves precision.

Chapter 2
Movement, Posture, and Gait:
The Good, the Bad, and the Ugly

We are what we repeatedly do.

—ARISTOTLE

As an athlete, you might stride, pedal, pull, row, or jump thousands of times in a single outing. Over time, these movements can create muscle imbalances and wear and tear on your joints, often resulting in injury. Likewise, your day-to-day movements, posture, and gait impact the integrity of your body. You can protect your body from prematurely wearing out by improving the quality of your movement. Pilates cross-training helps improve all of your movements, from the simplest to the most complex.

In this chapter you'll improve your body awareness, identify three types of movement, and explore the ABCs—criteria for creating good movement. You'll also look at posture and gait, since they are often the starting point for creating movement.

Learning Movement

As a child you may have learned sports by observing and imitating friends and other people who seemed to know what they were doing. As Richard A. Schmidt and Craig A. Wrisberg noted in their book, *Motor Learning and Performance*, along the way you passed through three stages of learning: cognitive, motor, and autonomous.

Cognitive learning is the choppy phase when you first tried to perform a movement. It's when you first fell off your bike, snowplowed for survival on green runs, or got shaky while climbing. Motor learning is the mastery phase. It's when you learned to race your bike against the wind, turn your skis on a dime, and scale cliffs like Spider-Man. The third stage is autonomous movement; it's the autopilot phase. You just do it! You entered "the zone," and your movements became smooth, seemingly effortless, and without thought.

As a baby you went through this same process when you learned to sit, stand, and walk. You persevered until what at first made you fall became easy and effortless. As you became an adult, these movements evolved further and were influenced by your level of awareness, alignment, fitness, and self-esteem. Likewise, in sports your ability to master new skills has been influenced by these factors.

Creating Awareness

Creating more awareness begins by noticing the way you move and feel in your body. Pay attention to how you move in your day-to-day activities and while practicing sports. Notice how you are sitting as you read this book. Are you slumped on a couch? Do you feel any tension in your body? A busy lifestyle with many roles and responsibilities can shortchange your mind-body connection. Many people slouch all day behind desks and crane their necks to see computers. At five o'clock they leave the office but remain in these postures. Next time you go for a run or a bike ride, notice your posture. Do you cycle with tense shoulders or hold your

breath while running? When finished, do you notice any aches or pains? Lack of awareness perpetuates poor movement that can lead to overuse injuries. Like a tree that is weakly rooted on a steep and sandy hillside, over time the whole structure gives way.

Right-Handed—Left-Footed

Noticing your side dominance is a quick and easy way to gain more awareness of your movements. Most people know if they're right-handed or left-handed, but do you know which foot you lead with when striding or pedaling? Test your awareness by answering the following questions:

- Which foot do you step with first when walking up stairs?

- Which shoulder do you prefer to sling a bag over?

- If sitting in a chair with someone directly behind you, which direction would you turn to look at her?

- When you talk on the phone, which ear do you hold to the receiver?

Many people use one side of their body to stabilize while the other side mobilizes. Right-handed people often stabilize with their left side while moving with their right side. For example, if I asked you to stand on one leg, which one would you choose? A righty is more likely to stand on his left leg. In athletes, dominant-side movements create muscle imbalances in strength and flexibility. While one side gets stronger, the other side gets weaker. Pilates cross-training won't make you ambidextrous, but it will improve your muscle balance.

Let's identify three types of movement.

Good Movement

Good movement flows. It's easy, energy efficient, and feels effortless. It requires the least amount of time and energy, thereby increasing ease and grace. It is done with the best possible alignment and uses gravity to its advantage. It is core centered, supported by the breath, and creates the least amount of wear and tear on the muscles and joints. Good movement embodies the six principles of Pilates: breathing, centering, concentration, control, fluid motion, and precision. Good movement begins with awareness.

Bad Movement

Bad movement stutters, stops, and starts, like a car that needs a tune-up. It requires more time, energy, and force, thereby increasing the work and strain on the muscles and joints. With bad movement, breathing is not coordinated with the movement, alignment is usually poor, and the core musculature does not assist in the movement.

Ugly Movement

Ugly movement is jerky and lacks control. Breathing is shallow, if not erratic. Tension and strain are noticeable while engaging in the activity. It is the kind of movement that makes us wince to observe. The limbs and torso seem to have no relationship in the execution of the movement, and the person seems to lack proper balance and coordination. Both bad and ugly movement can result from:

- Lack of awareness
- Poor technique
- Misalignments
- Muscle imbalances
- Insufficient core strength
- Previous injuries

All movement can be dramatically improved by practicing Pilates.

The ABCs of Good Movement

Now that you've improved your awareness of movement, let's consider three factors that influence your ability to create good movement: alignment, balanced muscles, and core-centered movement.

A = Alignment

Good movement begins with the proper alignment of your spine. Proper alignment enables you to freely bend, twist, flex, and extend. It improves your range of motion and also your balance. By stacking your spine, you honor its natural curves. As a result, your skeletal framework is better able to support you and your muscles can engage more evenly.

Proper alignment of your spine also improves the alignment of your hips, legs, and feet. As a result, you experience greater efficiency of movement and less wear and tear on your joints.

In the next section, Your Posture, we will address how to create proper alignment. By practicing Pilates you'll improve your alignment, and as a result, the quality of your movement as well.

No matter how well tuned a vehicle, if it is misaligned, the steering wheel will vibrate, the tires will wear unevenly, and other parts will be damaged. The same holds true for your body. Misalignment of your spine and limbs creates unnecessary tension in your neck, shoulders, back, and in other joints of your body. Misalignment reduces the range of motion of your joints and the quality of your breathing. It demands that your muscles work harder than necessary to do everything from standing to walking to practicing sports or Pilates.

When practicing Pilates, always maintain the best possible alignment and form. For example, when doing the Side-Kick Series, master stabilizing your torso before expanding the range of motion of your kicks, circles, and leg lifts. If you are practicing the Hundred, master the C-curl position before moving on to more difficult variations. Evaluate your progress and proficiency at each exercise in terms of your alignment first and your range of motion second. You will be less likely to injure yourself, and you will be rewarded with more core strength, muscle balance, and flexibility.

B = Balanced Muscles

Balanced muscles are strong, flexible, and resilient. They make everything from walking to skiing, cycling, and running easier. By balancing your muscles, you improve the integrity of your joints and their functioning.

To maintain joint integrity and alignment, the muscles must be balanced in strength and flexibility. Pilates creates balance by uniformly strengthening and stretching muscles. You can improve your muscle balance by creating a sense of oppositional energy. To better understand this concept, try this exercise. Hold your arms out to your sides at shoulder height and imagine that they are neon light tubes filled with light or energy from your shoulders all the way into your fingertips. Imagine that the light completely fills the tube. Notice what happens to the muscles of your arms. Do they feel more engaged front to back and inside and out? Apply the same technique to your legs. In doing so, you'll create gentle traction in your joints. You can also imagine that you are lengthening your limbs like octopus tentacles while keeping them firmly connected to your center. Create imaginary resistance as if you were under water.

C = Core-Centered Movement

Most people haven't begun to tap into their potential as athletes until they've developed a strong core. Core-centered movement improves range of motion, power, and balance. Integrating your core enables you to produce powerful movement. It is what connects the lower body to the upper body to create a dynamic line of energy. A kayaker who uses her core to power her stroke is core centered. A climber who utilizes his body tension to make a delicately balanced movement is core centered.

In addition, core strength helps to elongate and decompress the spine and joints. Movement that lacks a centered core can create compression in your spine and joints. Compression is like a traffic jam—stressful and unpredictable. One day you're skiing the bumps, and the next you're struggling to get out of a chair. Pilates gives you the freedom to enjoy your sports and eliminate "traffic jams" by improving core strength.

Movement, Posture, and Gait

15

MOVEMENT MATTERS

Your Posture

Posture sets the stage for the quality of your movements. It is determined largely by your alignment, muscle balance, and core strength. It has been said that how you do something is how you do everything. From that perspective, improving your posture is the simplest way to improve all of your movement. Good posture enables a swimmer to be more powerful, a cyclist to be more aerodynamic, and a runner to be faster and reduce stress on the joints.

We grow up with many misconceptions about posture. We are told to lift our chin, stick out our chest, and pull back our shoulders. Instead of creating better alignment, we look and feel like stiff wooden soldiers. What's the chance of producing fluid and good movement?

How we feel affects our posture and vice versa. Our movements and posture not only *reflect* but also *affect* our mental state and the elevation of our spirit. Imagine what your posture is saying to the person next to you right now. If we are sad or depressed, we are more likely to slouch and stand with our shoulders rounded and our head bowed forward. When we slouch, our internal organs get squished and are unable to function optimally. If we feel good, we are more likely to stand tall with our chest lifted. Good posture begins with good alignment.

The Sequoia Tree

Look at an old sequoia tree reaching skyward in Yosemite National Park. It has great alignment and great longevity. Sequoias grow to be more than 300 feet tall and can be more than 3,200 years old. Good alignment makes gravity a friend instead of an enemy.

Imagine your feet anchored into the ground like tree roots and the top of your head pulled magnetically toward the sky. Contrary to popular belief, standing tall is easier than slouching, because it requires less muscular effort.

Take a look at yourself in the mirror and notice a few things. Stand with your feet hip-width apart. Do you tilt your head to one side? Are your shoulders level? Do they roll forward? Notice if one arm hangs closer or longer by your side than the other. See if you can draw a vertical line from your collarbones to the front of your hip bones, down through the center of your kneecaps, to your third toes. Notice if your kneecaps face forward or if they roll inward or pull outward. Do you lock out your knees? Notice where you balance your weight over your feet. Do the front of your feet line up, or is one slightly forward of the other?

The following photos illustrate examples of good, bad, and downright ugly postures that we often find ourselves visiting in the course of a day. Where do you call home?

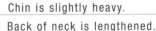
Good Posture

In this photo, notice the plumb line from the ears to the ankles. Weight is evenly distributed between both feet, which are about hip-width apart with the toes pointing forward. Kneecaps are in line with the hip bones. Legs are straight, yet the knees are soft. The hips are level, and the natural curves of the spine are honored. The ribs are soft and recede naturally into the chest, yet the chest is open. The shoulders are down and gently back, and the arms hang easily with the palms facing in toward the thighs. The back of the neck is lengthened and the chin is slightly heavy, yet level. The crown of the head floats up as if a string were pulling it.

Crown of the head floats up as if a string were pulling it.

Chin is slightly heavy.

Back of neck is lengthened.

The chest is open and collarbones reach outward.

Ribs are soft and recede.

Natural lumbar curve of spine is honored.

Arms hang easily by sides with palms facing in.

Knees are soft and not locked.

Feet are hip-width apart with kneecaps and toes pointed forward.

Bad Posture

In this photo, the low back is swayed, causing the pelvis to tip forward and the knees to lock. By swaying the lower back, the hip flexors tighten, the hamstrings become overstretched, and lower-back pain is likely to result. In addition, this posture puts pressure on the veins in the legs, thereby decreasing circulation and increasing stress on the soft tissues of the knees.

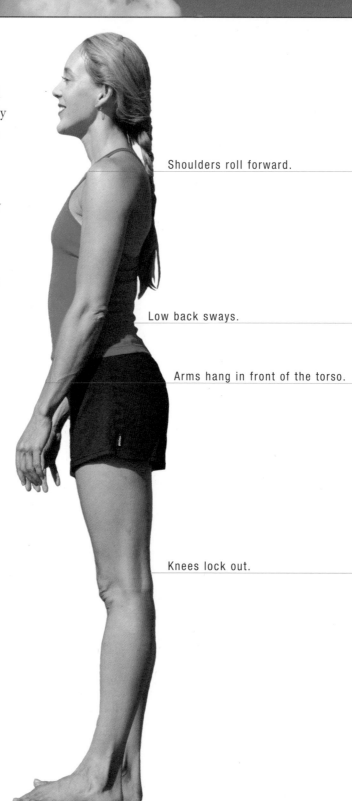

Shoulders roll forward.

Low back sways.

Arms hang in front of the torso.

Knees lock out.

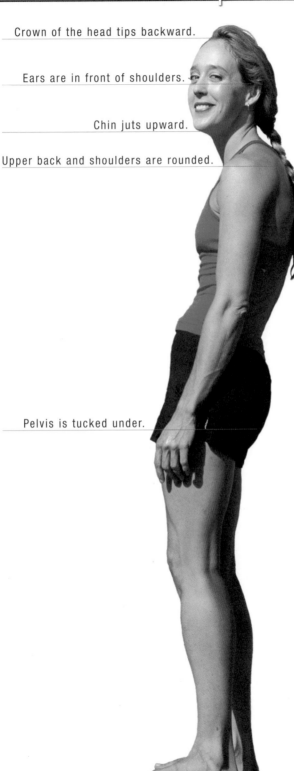

Crown of the head tips backward.

Ears are in front of shoulders.

Chin juts upward.

Upper back and shoulders are rounded.

Pelvis is tucked under.

Ugly Posture

In this photo, notice the shortening at the back of the neck and the rounding forward of the shoulders. This is referred to as "forward head posture." In the short term this posture can cause headaches, but over the course of a lifetime it can lead to dowager's hump and kyphosis. Also notice that the pelvis is tucked under, or tipped backward. This results in shortening of the hamstrings and lower abdominal muscles.

If you recognize yourself in either of the last two photos, work on correcting your posture before it's too late. The older we get, the stiffer and less articulate our joints become. If you've ever observed elderly people unable to stand upright, it is often because they've lost the mobility in their joints to do so. By practicing Pilates regularly, you'll not only become stronger and more flexible, you'll stand taller.

In addition to standing, we find ourselves in two other postures that influence the quality of our movement: lying down and sitting.

Movement, Posture, and Gait

19

MOVEMENT MATTERS

Lying Down Posture

Many Pilates exercises begin by lying down, therefore it is important to consider your alignment in this position. As you change your body's orientation to gravity, the principles of good alignment remain constant.

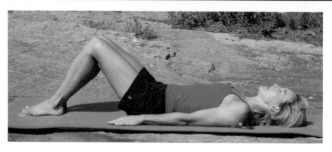

Lying on your back, bend your knees and bring your feet hip-width apart. Bring your shoulders down and back so that you feel your upper back making contact with the floor. Allow the front of your rib cage and sternum to be soft and recede into your spine. Slightly nod your chin toward your chest so that the back of your neck is lengthened. Keep a small space between the floor and the back of your neck. If the back of your head does not easily meet the floor but instead tips backward, place a pillow under your head to alleviate shoulder or neck tension and improve your alignment. Rock your pelvis forward and back until you reach a neutral position where your sacrum, the flat wedge-shaped bone at the base of your spine, feels heavy on the floor and you have approximately a finger's width of space beneath your low back. In this position your hip bones and pubic bones should be parallel to the floor. Pull your navel to your spine. If you are lying down with your legs out straight, apply the same alignment principles.

Seated Posture

Distribute your weight evenly between both of your sitz bones. These bones are part of your pelvis and can be felt by rocking back and forth on a hard surface while seated. Stack your spine as if there were a wall behind your back. Lengthen your waistline and tip your hips front to back until your pelvis is level and your lumbar curve is not flattened out or exaggerated. Draw your navel to your spine and open your chest. Bring your shoulder blades down and back as if you were gently squeezing a small ball under each arm. Lengthen the back of your neck and reach the crown of your head upward.

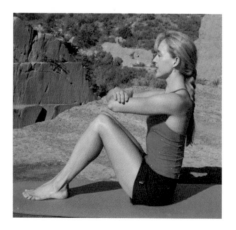

Your Gait

Have you ever recognized someone by the way she walks, even before you could see her face? Picture your mother or father and imagine how she or he walks. Now imagine a close friend of yours walking. Our posture, speed, and stride length make our gait as unique to us as our personality.

Similar to other movement, the quality of your gait affects the integrity of your joints. Conversely, the integrity of your body affects your gait. Poor alignment of the ankles, knees, and hips can result in injuries to the back, knees, hips, and feet. If one hip is rotated and slightly higher, such as in some forms of scoliosis, it creates a leg-length discrepancy affecting the knees as well. Like all movement, improving your gait begins with improving your alignment, muscle balance, and core strength. Let's define good, bad, and ugly gait. Please keep in mind that these are only guidelines and that everyone's gait is unique.

Good Gait

The biomechanics of good gait include pointing your feet forward so that your second toe is aligned with your kneecap. Ideally, you should strike through the outside of your heel and roll through to the inside of the ball of the foot. As you push off, the big toe should be the last to leave. By rolling from outside to inside, your foot can better absorb shock and propel you forward. As you transfer weight from one leg to the other, you should stay centered over your pelvis to minimize sway. Meanwhile, your arms and legs should move in opposition to allow your spine to rotate slightly. Your head should stay at approximately the same height while you stride.

Bad Gait

Bouncing up and down, swaying the hips side to side locking out the knees, and landing with force causes stress to the feet, knees, hips, and back. Exaggerated movements can cause the pelvis to drop more to one side than the other, creating misalignment of the knee and foot. In addition, the iliotibial band may tighten up in an effort to minimize rotation.

Bad gait can also be characterized by restricting movement in the hips and arms. Not allowing the pelvis to rotate freely can cause inappropriate rotation at the knee joint, leading to stress and injury. Likewise, keeping your arms rigid creates unnecessary stress in your shoulder joints and your spine.

Ugly Gait

Ugly gait builds upon bad gait and includes alignment issues such as forward-head posture and rounding the shoulders forward.

5 Tips for Improving Your Gait

1. As you stride, point your feet forward so your second toe is aligned with your kneecap.

2. Strike through the outside of your heels and push off with your big toes.

3. Minimize sway from right to left and stay centered over your hips.

4. Minimize bouncing up and down or locking your knees, and keep your head level.

5. Move your arms and legs in opposition.

Creating good movement is central to Pilates and athletics. To appreciate how your body creates good movement, it is important to develop a fundamental understanding of biomechanics. The next chapter serves as a crash course in biomechanics and will help you to understand how your muscles and bones work together to create movement.

Chapter 3

Know Your Gear:
Basic Biomechanics of Movement

*To every action,
there is an equal and opposite reaction.*

—ISAAC NEWTON

Do you know more about the dynamics of your skis and bindings than you do about your own body? If you're committed to improving the quality of your movement and maintaining a balanced body, it will serve you to develop a better understanding of basic biomechanics. Don't let the word scare you—biomechanics simply refers to how your bones, muscles, ligaments, and tendons work together to create movement.

This chapter provides a foundation for understanding basic biomechanics. Anatomy is included only so far as it helps to further your understanding. Our discussion is organized in the following order: the lower body, torso, and upper body. Since athletes typically begin movement from the feet, we'll begin with the lower body.

How you use your feet creates a ripple effect up your ankles, knees, hips, and spine. What impacts your spine affects the range of motion of your shoulders, neck, and head. It is important to note that we could begin this discussion from the top down as well. You propel yourself through space with your feet but lead with your eyes and head. Therefore the quality of your movement at either end affects your entire body. This chapter is not intended to be a primary reference, but instead will provide a foundation for discussion. If you suspect you have a biomechanical issue, please consult with an orthopedic doctor.

The Lower Body

Feet and Ankles

Since many outdoor athletics begin with the feet, improving foot strength, flexibility, and function go a long way toward preventing problems down the road. Faulty foot biomechanics can lead to injuries not only to the feet but also to the knees and hips. Bunions, iliotibial band tendonitis, patellar tendonitis, piriformis syndrome, sciatica, shin splints, and SI (sacroiliac) dysfunction can result from foot misalignments. Foot problems create muscle imbalances and place excess tension on the soft tissues of the joints. Likewise, the strength and flexibility of your legs, hips, and core impact how the foot functions.

The foot has 26 bones and two primary functions: to adapt to changing ground and to absorb shock. The feet have three points of contact that form a tripod: the ball of the big toe, the ball of the little toe, and the center of the heel bone. With the help of the ankles, your feet move in four directions (plantar flexion, dorsal flexion, eversion, and inversion), allowing you to easily adapt to the changing slope of a trail. Biomechanical problems include excessive pronation and supination.

Excessive Pronation: Excessive rolling inward of the foot toward the big toe places extra stress on the inside ligaments of the foot and creates ankle instability. It is also responsible for numerous injuries to the knees, hips, and back. Excessive foot pronation can be hereditary or may develop as a result of poor biomechanics. Poor choices in footwear such as high heels or flip-flops without arch support can exacerbate the problem. Strengthening the muscles of your feet and legs and using orthotics can provide support and improve foot function.

Excessive Supination: Often caused by tight ligaments and a high arch, excessive supination is when the foot is overly rigid and doesn't roll enough to the inside. Excessively supinating feet are unable to absorb shock. Shin splints, plantar fasciitis, and Achilles tendonitis can result. Sometimes a soft padded support placed inside the shoe along the arch is helpful. Strengthening and stretching the muscles of the feet and using custom orthotics often improve foot function.

A professional gait analysis is helpful to evaluate the biomechanics of your feet. However, a quick and dirty approach requires checking your running shoes. Place your shoes side by side on a table. If they tip inward, you overpronate. If they tip outward, you oversupinate.

Knees and Legs

Survey most athletes, and unequivocally you'd find knee injuries to be at the top of the injury list. According to *The Sports Injury Handbook*, "Nearly one million knee surgeries are performed each year in the United States." The knee is a hinge joint that primarily bends and extends the leg. Its junction is where the femur bone sits on top of the larger of the two lower leg bones, the tibia. Between these bones are two cushions of cartilage, called the meniscus. They provide support for your body weight over the knee joint. Over time, if uneven pressure is applied to the lower leg bones due to muscle imbalances and misalignments, the meniscus becomes compromised and the knees become arthritic.

The knee has four main stabilizing ligaments: the anterior and posterior cruciate ligaments and the medial and lateral collateral ligaments. Below the kneecap is the patellar tendon. It connects the kneecap to the shinbone. Alignment and muscle balance in the legs and hips helps maintain the integrity of your knees. Sports such as running and cycling create muscle imbalances that compromise the soft tissues of the knee. In an effort to create stability, the body begins working excessively from certain leg muscles. For example, an imbalance between the calves and shins may result in a tightening of the Achilles tendon and the creation of shin splints. Pilates helps you maintain proper muscle balance and alignment by uniformly stretching and strengthening your body.

The Torso

Think of your torso as a house. The pelvic muscles form the floor, the core muscles are the walls, and the diaphragm is the ceiling. The rib cage is the second story, and the spine is like a spiral staircase allowing you to move about your house.

Pelvis

Many athletes never give a thought to the position of their pelvis. As a result they often experience lower-back pain or injury. The pelvis sits on top of your femur bones like a bowl. It tips forward, back, and side to side. Its position impacts the alignment of your spine and lower body. For example, if you tip your pelvis forward so as to arch your lower back, your lower back tightens, your knees lock out, and your feet roll inward.

Envision your pelvis as a basin of water that tips forward, back, and side to side. While standing, tip your hips forward and back as if you were pouring water out the front and back of a basin. In other words, alternate between arching and flattening out your lower back by moving your pelvis. Now find a neutral position where no water is spilled and your pelvis is level. In this position, you should be able to draw a parallel line from your hip bones to your pubic bones. If you were lying down, these same lines would also be parallel with the floor. In this position you would have approximately a finger's width of space between your lower back and the floor. It is important to be able to move from one position to the other and also identify a neutral place in between.

The Abs Family

Have you ever been to a "core-conditioning" class where crunching your brains out was the name of the game? Works great for a six-pack, which is actually an eight-pack, but don't expect a stronger core. The reason is simple—crunching doesn't train the most important core muscle: the transverse abdominus (TA).

The abdominal muscles consist of four layers of muscle that provide stability and mobility:

- Rectus abdominus (the six-pack)

- External obliques (waistline muscles)

- Internal obliques (waistline muscles)

- Transverse abdominus (corset muscle)

The rectus abdominus (six-pack) is mainly used in flexion (sit-ups) and assists the other three muscles. It is the most superficial of the abdominal muscles and the least important for spinal support, movement, and breathing. The obliques assist in side bending, flexing, twisting, and engage during deep exhalations. The transverse abdominus (TA), the deepest layer of abdominal muscle, is the torso's primary core stabilizer for movement and spinal support.

The TA wraps around your waistline and, when engaged, acts like a corset, minimizing the width of your waist. The easiest way to engage your TA is to place your hands around your waist and cough. Engaging your abdominal girdle, or core, can be as simple as drawing your navel to your spine so that your waist narrows like an hourglass. Another way to think about engaging your core is to imagine that you are zipping up a tight pair of blue jeans fresh out of the dryer. Proper breathing that emphasizes expanding your lungs and rib cage while narrowing your midsection provides support for your spine, massages your organs, and improves your alignment.

The Spine

*If your spine is
inflexibly stiff at 30,
you are old;
if it is completely flexible
at 60,
you are young.*

—JOE PILATES

Anyone who's learned to drive a stick shift knows there's a critical difference between the clutch and the brake. Once you figure this out, you can drive fast or slow and, more important, smoothly. Articulating your spine is a lot like learning to drive a stick. It means doing many things at the same time, seamlessly. This is also true of any sport. To effectively integrate the individual parts of a Pilates movement into a whole requires moving your spine. Our spines consist of 26 articulating vertebrae and, when free, can sequence movement from top to bottom, bottom to top, and from both ends simultaneously. We have 7 cervical vertebrae (neck), 12 thoracic (upper back), 5 lumbar (lower back), a sacrum, and tailbone (coccyx). The sacrum is composed of five fused vertebrae and a coccyx, consisting of three or four fused vertebrae. This vertebral column has two functions: to move the torso and to protect the spinal column. The spine moves in four basic directions: flexion, extension, side bending, and rotation. Along with the TA, muscles known as the spinal extensors help you to maintain an upright posture, arch, side bend, and rotate your spine.

The spine has four curves (cervical, thoracic, lumbar, and sacral) that cushion the spinal cord and absorb shock as we move. We are born without a cervical or lumbar curve, but as we learn to crawl and walk, these curves develop. Each curve has a distinct range of motion due to the shape of the vertebrae and thickness of the intervertebral discs. Over time the spinal curves can become reduced or exaggerated, creating "compression" in between each vertebra. Common spinal deviations include:

Lordosis: An exaggerated curve of the lumbar spine known as swayback. This is often caused by a weak core and tight hip flexors that cause the pelvis to drop forward. It results in compression and pain in the lower back.

Kyphosis: Also known as humpback, kyphosis is characterized by an exaggerated curve of the upper spine. Kyphosis shows itself as excessive rounding of the upper spine and a chest that caves inward. A person with kyphosis has difficulty standing upright and lying down flat without the aid of a pillow. Straightening the arms overhead may not only be uncomfortable but damaging to the shoulder's rotator cuff. This is because kyphosis limits the range of motion in the spine, which in turn limits the range of motion in the shoulders.

Scoliosis: A lateral curve in the spine that causes the vertebrae to bend and rotate, scoliosis can be structural or functional. Structural scoliosis is caused by genetic factors causing one side of the spine to grow faster than the other, whereas functional scoliosis is caused by dysfunctional movement patterns that affect the muscles but do not alter the structure of the spine. Functional scoliosis can result from poor posture or repeated unbalanced activity such as carrying a heavy backpack on one shoulder all the time. An easy way to see if scoliosis is structural or functional is to bend forward and have someone look at your spine. If the lateral curve disappears while standing, then it is most likely a functional scoliosis; if it remains, it is most likely structural.

The quality of your breath, posture, movement, and muscle balance plays a large role in maintaining the integrity of your spine. Tight hamstrings can cause the lumbar curve to flatten, whereas tight quadriceps and hip flexors can cause it to excessively arch, leading to swayback, also known as lordosis. Tight or weak neck and shoulder

muscles can compromise the cervical and thoracic curves. When the spine loses its natural curve, injuries such as herniated or bulging discs, slipped discs, pinched nerves, and sciatica can result. Pilates helps you maintain strong flexible muscles and improves the integrity of your spine.

Rib Cage

You have 12 ribs on either side of your rib cage protecting your lungs. Between each rib are intercostal muscles that lengthen and contract as you breathe. As you inhale, the ribs swivel up and outward like venetian blinds. As you exhale, the ribs swivel down and inward, decreasing the circumference of the rib cage. Over time, shallow breathing can cause these muscles to become inflexible and tight. Pilates breathing helps to regain the strength and flexibility of these muscles.

Diaphragm

The diaphragm is your primary muscle for breathing. It is a domelike muscle that attaches at the bottom of your lungs forming a ceiling between your powerhouse and rib cage. As you inhale and air is drawn into the lungs, the diaphragm drops down and outward. As you exhale, the diaphragm billows upward into your chest like a hot air balloon. This causes the abdominal muscles to be drawn inward and slightly upward. Proper movement of the diaphragm is required to maximize lung capacity and achieve optimal muscle endurance.

The Upper Body

Shoulder Girdle

The shoulder girdle is what makes a wide array of arm movements possible, and it has the greatest range of motion in the body. It consists of the breastbone, collarbones, and shoulder blades. The breastbone is the junction where the collarbones and ribs connect into the front of the body. The collarbones (clavicles) are two flat S-shaped bones that extend from the breastbone to the shoulder blades. They are commonly broken when falling on an outstretched arm. The shoulder blades (scapulae) are two triangular-shaped bones that lie flat against your rib cage. They slide over the ribs, moving up (elevation), down (depression), forward (protraction), and back (retraction). They roll easily through a combination of these movements. The muscles relied upon to create these movements include the rhomboids, levator scapulae, trapezius, and serratus anterior.

With all its potential for movement, the shoulder has only one true joint: the sterno-clavicular joint. No wonder shoulder injuries are so common. Shoulder movement happens at four junctions. All four must work together for the shoulder to function properly. See if you can feel them in your own body.

1. **Sterno-clavicular:** Between the breastbone and collarbones.
2. **Acromio-clavicular:** Between the lateral edge of the collarbone and shoulder blade.
3. **Gleno-humeral:** The shallow dishlike socket where the upper arm bone connects into the shoulder. This is a place of tremendous mobility.
4. **Scapulo-thoracic:** The place where the shoulder blade and rib cage make contact.

Maintaining the integrity of the shoulder is a small band of muscles known as the rotator cuff. The rotator cuff muscles, also known as SITS muscles (supraspinatus, infraspinatus, terres minor, and subscapularis), add stability and keep the upper-arm bone (humerus) in the shoulder socket. They make it possible to lift your arms overhead. You can strengthen these muscles by doing exercises that internally and externally rotate the upper-arm in the shoulder socket. In addition, strengthening the rhomboids, trapezius, and serratus anterior adds to the integrity of the shoulder. Muscle imbalances often lead to one of two common injuries: shoulder dislocation and shoulder impingement.

According to the National Center for Health Statistics, in 2003 approximately 13.7 million people went to the doctor's office for a shoulder problem. Athletes engaging in sports where reaching repeatedly overhead is required, such as swimming, climbing, and kayaking, are more likely to injure their shoulders. If you suffer from a stiff shoulder, experience pain, or feel as though your shoulder could slide out of its socket, see an orthopedic doctor for an assessment. Shoulder injuries can be tedious to heal, and it's easy to make the problem worse without a qualified assessment.

Being able to differentiate the movements of the shoulders and the arms helps maintain healthy shoulders and influence the alignment of your spine. If I asked you to raise your arms to shoulder height, what do your shoulders do? If you are able to differentiate, then your shoulders stay down and uninvolved. If your shoulders creep up and your chest falls, draw your shoulder blades down your back toward your spine and lift your sternum so your collarbones broaden and your chest opens. Slide your shoulder blades down your back into imaginary pockets, similar to the movement you make when sliding your hands into jean pockets. Engage the muscles below and behind your armpits as if you were squeezing tiny pillows under your arms. Doing so helps to release tension in your neck and shoulders and maintains the integrity of your shoulder joint. Now raise your arms over your head. Are you wearing

your shoulders like earrings or are you busy yanking them down? Neither is optimal. A healthy range of motion means allowing your shoulder blades to rotate outward and upward from your spine.

The Arms

The arm consists of the upper-arm bone (humerus) and large and small lower-arm bones: the ulna and the radius. The primary muscles used to move the arm include the deltoids, pectoralis major, latissimus dorsi (lats), triceps, and biceps.

The elbow is primarily a hinge joint. A second joint, located where the humerus and radius meet, allows rotation of the forearm. The elbow has two important ligaments: one on the inside (the medial collateral ligament) and one on the outside (the lateral collateral ligament). Together, these ligaments connect the upper arm to the lower arm and provide elbow stability. Muscle imbalances between the flexors and extensors can compromise the integrity of these ligaments and lead to elbow tendonitis.

The Hands

The human hand contains 27 bones: the wrist accounts for 8, the palm contains 5, and the remaining 14 are finger bones. The muscles that bend and straighten the fingers and wrist attach into tendons at the elbow. On the way they pass through a bony archway at the wrist called the carpal tunnel. Excessive bending at the wrist can cause inflammation of these tendons and lead to numbness in the thumb and index finger. Injuries to the hands and fingers from sports such as rock climbing often result from contracting muscles for too long, twisting or side bending of the fingers, and muscle imbalances between the flexor and extensor muscles. Many times the flexors become stronger than the extensors, leading to elbow tendonitis.

Neck and Head and Eyes

On average the human head weighs a whopping eight pounds. That's a lot of weight resting on your shoulders. The head sits on top of the spine on an axis and tips front to back like a seesaw and side to side like a disc. It also tips and tilts while rotating—like a Tilt-a-Whirl. When properly aligned, your head sits over your shoulders. Long hours slouched behind a computer, whiplash, long-distance cycling, rock climbing, and a weak core can all compromise the alignment of your head and neck. A slight misalignment can impact your entire spine and lead to conditions known as forward head posture, dowager's hump, and kyphosis.

Forward Head Posture (FHP): FHP occurs when the head moves forward, the torso rounds backward, and the hips tip forward to compen-

sate. The natural curve of your cervical and lumbar spine becomes diminished. A lack of stability in the neck pulls your entire spine out of alignment. FHP places excessive stress on the cervical spine, causing head and neck aches, temporomandibular joint diseases (TMJ) and disorders of the jaw, shortness of breath, and mid- and low-back pain. Experts say that for every inch your head is in front of your ears, it adds an additional 10 pounds of extra work to the neck and upper-back muscles. FHP can also create dowager's hump or kyphosis. You may notice FHP in yourself or others. Signs include rounded upper back and shoulders, ears in front of the shoulders, and chin jutting upward.

Dowager's Hump: To compensate for neck instability created by conditions such as FHP or injuries to the neck, the body may produce a lump on the backside of the neck between the shoulders, known as dowager's hump. This clump of cartilage functions to create stability for the cervical spine.

If you suspect your head is misaligned, have a friend evaluate your side-profile posture. Ideally, she should be able to draw an imaginary line from your ear to your shoulder to your hip, knee, and ankle. Have her estimate how many inches your ears are in front of your shoulders.

You can improve the alignment of

your head and your entire spine by where you focus your eyes. The adage "keep your eye on the ball" applies. If you practice good posture but focus your eyes downward, before you know it you'll be rounding your shoulders forward and sinking your chest. For more tips on better posture, please refer to Chapter 2.

Chapter 4

Self-Assessment:
What's the Body Got to Say?

The unexamined life is not worth living for man.

—SOCRATES

We spend an enormous amount of time studying the techniques of our sports and reading up on the latest gear. We end up knowing more about the gearshifts on our bikes than we do about our bodies. The self-assessment test in this chapter addresses this knowledge imbalance. It considers five criteria of fitness that are improved upon by practicing Pilates. They are core strength, flexibility and range of motion, uniform muscle balance, movement skills, and a mind-body connection. Each provides a link in a chain strengthened through Pilates cross-training. The self-assessment test is designed to help you determine which links need the most work. By balancing all five links, you'll improve your odds of staying injury free, performing your best, and maintaining longevity as an athlete.

The Criteria

1 Core Strength: Your "Powerhouse"

Core strength refers to the muscles of your abdominals, lower back, and hips. Tapping into core strength is an inside job. You don't do a sit-up to tap into it; you exhale deeply and pull your navel to your spine. Core strength enables you to elongate and support your spine, execute movement with power, and maintain a strong sense of balance.

Flexing, extending, side bending, and twisting your spine require engaging your core. Without core support, excessive stress is placed on your spine, hips, knees, and ankles. Core strength makes your movements more powerful. A weak core is like a heavy bag of potatoes that your arms and legs work hard to haul around. A strong core connects the upper and lower body and transmits power from one end to the other. Like a guitar string that is tuned and tight, a strong core creates a line of energy through the body. Tightening your core as you press through your feet creates a line of energy from your center out through your head. It's what gives power to a karate punch. It's what enables a climber to maintain body tension while rock climbing and a paddler to create a powerful stroke. Likewise, it's what helps a skier pack more power behind her turns and, in the process, minimize load on her knees.

Core strength also improves your balance. Since your center of balance resides two inches below the belly button and one inch in front of your spine, engaging core muscles makes it easier to stand on one leg and balance. If you've ever seen someone walk a slack line or tightrope, chances are good they are engaging their core. Next time you're feeling slightly off balance, pull your navel to your spine.

2 Flexibility and Range of Motion

True flexibility can be achieved only when all muscles are uniformly developed.

—JOE PILATES

Flexibility is what allows a joint to move freely through its designed range of motion. Watch little kids play; they stretch and bend themselves like doughy unbaked pretzels. Being flexible allows you to stretch, flex, and curl and to extend your spine and limbs easily.

There are two types of flexibility: static and dynamic. Static flexibility is required for proper range of motion around a joint. Dynamic flexibility is required for movements that are fast and powerful, such as leaping. Maintaining a stem position while climbing requires static flexibility. Lifting the leg into the stem position requires dynamic flexibility.

Flexibility can be measured on a continuum that ranges from hyperflexible to completely inflexible. Hyperflexible athletes tend to be women. Examples of hyperflexibility include locking out the knees and elbows. These athletes benefit from increased stability around the joint and redefining a safe range of motion. Excessive flexibility can lead to joint instability.

Most people are more flexible in some muscles than others. For example, an athlete with very flexible hamstrings may have very tight quadriceps and hip flexors. If you find yourself on the inflexible end of the continuum, take the time to stretch. Joints are designed to move. Inarticulation leads to loss of range of motion, calcium buildup, and arthritis. Observe an elderly person who has trouble standing upright, and you'll understand what permanent loss of joint range of motion looks like. Don't let this happen to you.

No matter what your age or level of flexibility, your body *always* benefits from stretching. Stretching improves circulation, removes toxins, improves the elasticity and resiliency of your muscles and joints, and improves your posture. In addition, stretching is good for your back. By improving flexibility you'll decrease your chances of experiencing low-back pain. Flexible muscles mean better range of motion for your joints. Maintaining flexible muscles reduces the risk of injury to the knees.

3 Uniform Muscle Balance

Muscle balance is required for the integrity of your joints. Our sports, lifestyle, posture, gait, and any movement that is repetitive can contribute to muscle imbalances. Muscle imbalances leave our joints screaming, "Pay attention to me before I get ripped away from your kneecap!" Tendons, the very things holding muscles to bones, get pulled and tugged as if a war is going on between opposing forces within your body. The two teams are the "agonists" and the "antagonists." While one pulls (contracts), the other stretches (lengthens). Problems arise when one team is always lengthening and the other team is always shortening. One day you make a simple move you've made thousands of times before, only this time the rope breaks. Like any healthy relationship, there has to be give and take.

Most sport-specific injuries are caused by muscle imbalances that developed over time. The narrower your focus on one or two types of athletics, the higher your risk of creating muscle imbalances. The more sports in which you regularly participate, the less likely you are to have major muscle imbalances. Pilates develops the body evenly, front to back, top to bottom, and side to side. Uniform muscle balance is obtained by improving the flexibility of overused muscles and the strength of underused muscles.

The following is a list some of the major muscles in which athletes experience imbalances.

LOCATION	FRONT SIDE (Anterior)	BACK SIDE (Posterior)
Wrist and Hand	Flexors	Extensors
Forearm	Flexors	Extensors
Upper Arm	Biceps	Triceps
Torso	Pectorals	Trapezius and Rhomboids
Torso	Abdominal Muscles	Spinal Extensors
Hips	Hip Flexors	Hip Extensors
Upper Leg	Quadriceps	Hamstrings
Lower Leg	Shins	Calves

4 Movement Skills

Good movement requires minimal time and energy, thereby increasing ease and grace and decreasing wear and tear on the muscles and joints. In addition, good movement requires awareness, control, and precision. A lack of good movement perpetuates muscle imbalances and inflexibility.

One of the greatest things you can do to improve at your sport is to improve your movement skills. For example, how is your posture? Do you stand up tall like a sequoia? What about your gait? Do you bounce or sway when you walk? The higher your quality of movement, the more enjoyable your sport, the less likely you are to be injured, and the more likely you will be athletic into your golden years.

5 Mind-Body Connection

Do you get into the "zone" when working out, or do you simply "zone out"? In other words, how's your mind-body connection? You're more likely to get injured on days when you feel less connected to your body.

A strong mind-body connection increases clarity of thought, improves quality of movement, and elevates enjoyment of your sport. A strong mind-body connection helps you make more-intuitive decisions regarding the best way to solve a problem.

One of the reasons we love our sports is because they focus our energy and give us a break from the rest of life. When you ride, ski, or bike, do you find yourself distracted by thoughts beyond what you're doing? It's in the now that we make our greatest discoveries about life and ourselves.

In addition to lack of focus, we weaken our mind-body connection with excessive pressure on ourselves to perform. Life is full of pressure and expectations. We all know how it makes us feel: stressed. Putting too much pressure on yourself in athletics makes listening to your body impossible. In most cases prior to an injury, the body sends us multiple messages. An athlete's ability to stay connected while engaged in athletics is critical to avoiding injury.

A strong mind-body connection requires concentration and focus. Your Pilates practice will help you cultivate these skills. Make a commitment to yourself not to "zone out" or think about other things when doing your routine. The imagery provided for each exercise will help you visualize the movements you aim to create. Research shows that almost all world-class athletes use visualization to achieve peak levels of performance. Being able to see something with your mind's eye is tantamount to producing it in your body. As you learn Pilates, utilize the images provided. Avoid focusing on a particular muscle group; instead focus on images. Images create global changes in the body and strengthen the mind-body connection. For example, if you imagine your head being pulled up by a string, it affects the

entire spine, but if you stretch the back of your neck, only your neck is affected. Visualization creates the most efficient neuromuscular action in the body. It will help you create precise, flowing movements that are energy efficient and build strength and flexibility.

Your breathing has a significant effect on your ability to stay connected. Patterns such as holding your breath or hyperventilating can affect you adversely. Make certain that you are using your breath to set the rhythm of the Pilates exercise and that the exercise is helping you to breathe more deeply. By coordinating your breath and your movement, you will deepen your mind-body connection. By inhaling through the nose and exhaling through the mouth you'll stay dialed-in to your heart rate and exertion levels, dehydrate less quickly, and, because nose breathing stimulates the parasympathetic nervous system, you'll feel calmer. By tuning in to your body, you will cultivate and strengthen a mind-body connection that translates easily into your athletic endeavors.

Personal Assessment Test—Improve Your Awareness

In the middle of difficulty lies opportunity.

—ALBERT EINSTEIN

The following self-assessment test utilizes a paradigm known as the SWOT analysis. The SWOT analysis was developed by the Stanford Research Institute and identifies strengths, weaknesses, opportunities, and threats. Companies use it to create solid action plans for improvement and growth. Using a SWOT analysis, you can set realistic and achievable goals and create a plan empowering you to define your own Pilates routines to maximize results.

In this assessment you'll identify your greatest strength, weakness, opportunity, or threat. After completing the test, you'll want to consider any past injuries that you need to keep in mind when creating a plan of action. From this assessment you'll gain valuable insight into reducing your risk of injury, improving your performance, and maintaining your longevity as an athlete. Once you understand your strengths, weaknesses, opportunities, and threats, you'll be able to set reasonable, achievable long-term goals and create intermediate goals to measure your progress. Use the following worksheet to record current assessments. It's best to read to the question once, then answer with the first response that comes to mind. I recommend making a few photocopies of the assessment so that you can repeat the test in three months. Allow yourself 20 minutes of uninterrupted time to complete the test.

SWOT Analysis for Outdoor Athletes

Use the scale of 0–5 to answer the following test.

0 = Always
1 = 80 percent of the time
2 = 60 percent of the time
3 = 40 percent of the time
4 = 20 percent of the time
5 = Never

I. Core Strength

1. I experience low-back pain during or after doing my sport. _____

2. I often go a week without any specific core-strengthening activity. _____

3. I have difficulty with dynamic movement that requires speed and power. _____

4. I lose my balance easily. _____

5. I avoid push-ups, either because they are difficult or because they make my lower back hurt. _____

6. If I do an abdominal plank for one minute, my lower back arches and it feels like I am straining my back. _____

7. I find sit-ups and crunches to be strenuous. _____

8. If I stand on one leg and push up to the ball of my foot, I lose my balance within 30 seconds. _____

9. I could use more power in my sport. _____

10. I could improve my alignment by strengthening my midsection. _____

II. Flexibility and Range of Motion

11. I often go a week without stretching. _____

12. I consider myself fairly inflexible. _____

13. I find it difficult to sit with my legs out straight and touch my toes. _____

14. I find it uncomfortable to sit cross-legged (Indian-style) on the floor. _____

15. I have tight iliotibial bands. I experience pain on the outside of my knee and/or hip after my sport. _____

16. It is difficult to bring my arms over my head, keep them straight, and touch my palms together. _____

17. I have experienced muscle pulls or cramps. _____

18. I feel tension in my neck when I turn it side to side, left to right, or bow it down and up. _____

19. I have tight calves. _____

20. I have tight hamstrings. It's tough to touch my toes while keeping my legs straight. _____

III. Uniform Muscle Balance

21. I often go a week without any cross-training exercise. _____

22. In a typical season, I focus primarily on one sport. _____

23. I engage in my sport three or more days a week. _____

24. I engage in my sport three or more days in a row. _____

25. When I engage in my sport, I push myself to the point of exhaustion. _____

26. The day after participating in my sport, I feel stiff and achy in my joints. _____

27. I have had surgery due to an overuse injury. _____

28. I have experienced an overuse injury that required taking time off from my sport. _____

29. I tend to prefer sports that utilize the same major muscle groups (for example, running, skiing, and biking versus climbing and kayaking). _____

30. When I wave my arm, the back side of my upper arm jiggles like Jell-O. _____

IV. Movement Skills

31. I feel that my technique for my sport could use improvement. _____

32. I experience or have experienced sports injuries to my joints as a result of my sport. _____

33. After doing my sport, my knees, hips, or lower back hurt. _____

34. My shoulders and neck get tense from doing my sport. _____

35. My movements feel jerky and uncoordinated. _____

36. My reaction time is too long when encountering obstacles;
    could use more agility. _____

37. I often slouch or stand with less than ideal posture. _____

38. Even if I'm tired or sore, I force myself to do my sport. _____

39. I have difficulty pacing myself properly and run out of gas quickly. _____

40. My body is tired before my mind is ready to quit for the day. _____

V. Mind-Body Connection

41. When I engage in my sport, I am very competitive and sometimes risk
    injury before backing off. _____

42. While doing my sport, I am often tense and put too much pressure on
    myself to perform. _____

43. I have a hard time visualizing the movements I need to make to be energy
    efficient and solve problems quickly. _____

44. I consider myself to have a high tolerance for pain and often don't feel pain
    until I've done some damage. _____

45. I continue to do my sport even when I am injured or suspect
    an injury is developing. _____

46. While doing my sport, I am easily distracted by other people and
    things in my environment. _____

47. I have difficulty concentrating on one thing at a time. _____

48. While doing my sport, I spend a lot of time preoccupied with other things. _____

49. I hyperventilate when under stress. _____

50. I hold my breath and find myself frequently out of breath when
    doing my sport. _____

Identify Your Greatest Opportunity

After answering all 50 questions, place your scores in the five columns of the worksheet at the end of this chapter, then total your scores at the bottom of each column. The category that receives the highest score will be considered your strongest link. The category that receives the lowest score will be considered your weakest link and also your greatest opportunity. Any category with a zero will be considered a threat.

Other Considerations

In addition to your score, there are other areas that may impact your training. Some of them are addressed here and should be considered when developing an action plan in Chapter 5.

Stress

Consider the amount of stress in your life. Have you experienced a sudden change in health, lifestyle, stress, or training? Have you recently moved, switched jobs, gotten married or divorced? Too much stress combined with not enough rest and a poor diet do not allow the body to regenerate cells and maintain optimum health. Ask yourself the following questions as indicators of your level of stress:

- How often have you been sick in the past year?

- How are you sleeping: soundly or restlessly?

- How is your energy level?

- Have you experienced a change in your weight?

- How is your skin tone?

- Are you frequently irritable or tired?

Past and Present Injuries

Taking time off from the sports we love due to injuries is heavy on the spirit. By committing to a consistent cross-training practice, you'll reduce your chances of experiencing chronic injuries and maintain your longevity as an athlete. If you are currently dealing with even a slight injury, treat it with care. The tweaked shoulder or mild ache in your elbow may not seem like a big deal now, but it might be in the future. Twinges, burning sensation, joint stiffness, and swelling are your body's way of saying it has issues. If you are to learn from your injuries, you must identify their causes and reevaluate your training routines, adding cross-training to strengthen underdeveloped areas. By understanding how you incurred an injury and considering how you can avoid future injuries, you reduce the potential for them to become chronic. Even an injury that seems to occur suddenly may have been in the making for some time. Take a moment to answer yes or no to the following questions:

- Do you think you overtrain?

- If injured, do you continue to train anyway?

- Do you consider yourself to have a high threshold for pain?

- Once you feel better, do you resume the same level of training you practiced prior to the injury?

- Do you have an injury that has reoccurred or become chronic?

If you answered yes to all five questions, it is critical that you evaluate how you got injured in the first place, create a program that addresses those factors, and commit to a cross-training routine.

One Size Doesn't Fit All

As a general rule, men tend to benefit from additional flexibility training while women tend to benefit from more strength training. But as I mentioned before, we are all very good at training to our strengths and avoiding our weak links. Your gender, genetics, age, level of activity, occupation, and health all affect your physical makeup. While both men and women experience sports-related injuries due to overtraining, some injuries are more common in one gender or the other.

Two Eyes are Better Than One

In addition to taking this self-assessment, consider having an evaluation done by a qualified Pilates or fitness instructor who specializes in working with athletes.

Now that you've defined your SWOT and considered other factors that impact your training, Chapter 5 will help you create a plan.

Personal Assessment

Date:_____

CORE STRENGTH	FLEXIBILITY & R.O.M.	UNIFORM MUSCLE BALANCE	MOVEMENT SKILLS	MIND-BODY CONNECTION
1.	11.	21.	31.	41.
2.	12.	22.	32.	42.
3.	13.	23.	33.	43.
4.	14.	24.	34.	44.
5.	15.	25.	35.	45.
6.	16.	26.	36.	46.
7.	17.	27.	37.	47.
8.	18.	28.	38.	48.
9.	19.	29.	39.	49.
10.	20.	30.	40.	50.

TOTALS   Greatest Link: (Highest Score)   _____

Weakest Link: (Lowest Score)   _____

Identify Major Stresses in Your Life: _____

_____

_____

Identify Past or Current Injuries: _____

_____

_____

Chapter 5

Your Vision:
Cross-Training Goals

Begin with an End in Mind.

—STEPHEN COVEY

You would not go on a road trip without first deciding where to go. Similarly, you should begin your Pilates cross-training knowing what you want to accomplish. You vision and the extent to which you own it determine your destination and your chances of reaching it. Define the scope of your journey. Will it be long and far-reaching or will you stay close to home? Your vision reflects your values and makes every choice easier because you know what you want to accomplish. Do you value going for long runs in the morning or playing on the ski slopes with your kids? Would you like to run a marathon next year? Do you want to be touring the Rocky Mountains on your bicycle when you're 60 or backpacking in Canyonlands National Park when you're 80? What would you like to accomplish this month, next year, and for the rest of your life? Maybe your vision is as simple as enjoying a better quality of life today. Maybe you're interested in strengthening your core to alleviate back pain. Maybe you'd like to be able to touch your toes again. Like the headlamps on your car, your vision is what guides you forward when everything else is beyond sight.

Once you have a clear vision, it's time to set realistic and achievable goals and create a plan of action. To really create momentum, your goals need to be relevant and motivating. Take responsibility for where you are today in your fitness and make the decision to be proactive—commit to change. As you set out on your journey to greater personal fitness and well-being, it's important not only to know where you want to go but how you intend to get there. In other words, have a map.

Your Map

Your plan of action is a road map to navigate your fitness journey. The map consists of your final destination (long-term goals), landmarks (short-term goals), and a few mile markers (benchmarks) along the way. The directions on your map include:

Do It Today!:
Daily action to maximize your greatest opportunity
Weekly Pilates Routine:
Target your weakest links
Pay the Toll:
One thing you're willing to forgo to achieve your vision
Mile Markers:
Measure progress at 6 and 12 weeks

Do It Today!

To make change happen, you must take action immediately and regularly. Identify one thing to do every day that would pay a huge dividend toward achieving your vision. For example, if you want to gain more hamstring flexibility, commit to doing five minutes of gentle stretching every day. Maybe you want to improve your posture. Commit to slouching less at the computer or while driving. It doesn't have to be the same action each day, but it does have to be directed toward maximizing your greatest opportunity. In other words, turn your weakest link into your secret weapon.

Weekly Pilates Routine

Growing up, my brothers and I found our dad's fitness regimen to be like clockwork. He got up at the same time every morning. Tuesdays and Thursdays he swam; Mondays, Wednesdays, and Fridays he ran. He did core-conditioning exercises on his swimming days, stretched on his running days, and rested on Saturdays and Sundays. Today my father is a very fit and active 60-year-old who has maintained his longevity as an athlete.

Routines don't have to be this regimented, but they do require discipline. You don't have to always run the same trails or do the same Pilates exercises. Mix it up, be creative, have fun! Maybe you already know that you need more flexibility, but did you know you could benefit from improved movement skills as well? As you get into your routine, you'll want to add and change the exercises along the way. The routines found in Part III serve as a guide. I encourage you to create new routines or add new exercises to help you maximize your opportunity.

Before you commit to your routine, consider what time will be required and build it into your schedule. It is a fact that people who exercise first thing in the morning are less likely to have their routines interrupted than those who exercise after work. Whenever you do it is fine, just make sure it's an unbroken commitment to yourself. Keep your goals in sight and you'll be more motivated to stay disciplined. Posting a motivational photo or phrase in a place where you'll see it daily will reinforce your vision. Your Pilates cross-training will pay the biggest dividends if you are consistent and practice three to five times per week.

Occasionally, someone will ask me how long he or she should continue doing Pilates. I answer, "For as long as you value being active, strong, and flexible." Would you stop brushing your teeth after going to the dentist and having them cleaned and polished? Consistency is vital; don't wait until you have an injury to commit to a cross-training routine. Conversely, don't stop practicing because your injury is resolved. Be proactive about your fitness—commit to owning your body for the rest of your life. Your routine will change and evolve as you do. By practicing Pilates regularly, you will never be dependent on a gym or fitness trainer. Your routine is completely portable, adaptable, and free, 24/7.

Pay the Toll

Your journey is going to cost you 15 minutes a day, three to five times a week, and a proportional amount of energy. At a maximum, you'll have invested one hour and 15 minutes per week. Imagine what you'll gain in exchange. Consider what activity

you will have to forgo daily to do so. What's 15 minutes a day less TV or Internet surfing if it keeps you moving and enjoying your life? It's a small price to pay. Remember that nothing is free—you either pay a little now or a lot more later, in the form of injuries and pain. Consider it the price of admission to better fitness and athletic longevity.

Mile Markers

Setting 6- and 12-week mile markers (benchmarks) will make your commitment to change real. Mile markers should focus on improving your greatest opportunity, and therefore your weakest link. They should be quantifiable and specific. A 12-week mile marker might include improving your hamstring flexibility by 50 percent. To measure your current flexibility, stand on the floor with your legs straight and together. Keep your spine straight as you bend forward. Now measure the distance from your fingers to the floor. If the distance is currently four inches, then your 12-week benchmark would be two inches. Your mile markers should be relevant and keep you on track so you reach your final destination.

Use the following worksheet to create your map. I recommend making a few photocopies of the worksheet so that you can see where you are at regular intervals.

Your Map

I. Define Your Destinations—Know Where You Want to Go and Why

1. Final Destination: My lifetime vision as an outdoor athlete is: _____

_____

2. It is important to me for the following reasons: _____

_____

3. Landmark: Next year I want to accomplish: _____

_____

4. Mile Marker #1: In 6 weeks I would like to accomplish: _____

_____

5. Mile Marker #2: In 12 weeks I would like to accomplish: _____

_____

II. Landmarks: Define Your Best Route

6. I am committed to turning the following weak link into my greatest opportunity:_____

_____

_____

7. The one thing I will do consistently and daily to strengthen my weakness is: _____

_____

8. I am committed to doing my Pilates cross-training program _____ times per week.

9. I will sacrifice the following thing in order to accomplish my goal: _____

_____

III. Mile Markers (Benchmarks)

10. Six-Week Mile Marker: By the following date _____, I will accomplish the following:

_____

11. Twelve-Week Mile Marker: By the following date _____, I will accomplish the following:

_____

_____

Evaluate Your Progress

At 6 weeks and 12 weeks, if you've achieved your mile markers, congratulate yourself. Then begin the work of reevaluating your goals and setting new markers. I recommend continuing to set them at 6- and 12-week increments.

If you did not reach your mile markers, it's important to evaluate and learn from what went wrong. Sometimes the goals we set for ourselves are the equivalent of saying we want to drive from New York to Los Angeles in four hours. We are so eager to get somewhere that we risk never arriving at all. Begin by asking yourself the following questions:

- Did you create a compelling destination?

- Did you follow through on doing one thing every day?

- Did you set realistic and achievable mile markers?

- Did you pay the toll by making a sacrifice?

- What roadblocks did you allow to get in your way?

- Did you practice your routine regularly?

- Did you make it fun, or did it become a chore?

Remember: The only failure is in not recognizing what went wrong and acting to fix it. Recognize that you may need to change your approach and begin again. Keep in mind that the longer you persist with your Pilates practice, the more crossover you will experience in the quality of your sports and your life.

Your training program is ultimately effective when you are able to transfer the work you have done as an athlete to benefit the rest of your life.

Enjoy Your Journey

The road is better than the end.

—CERVANTES

Don't be in too big of a hurry to get where you're going. Take your time; enjoy where you are in this very moment. Appreciate all you've done thus far to get where you are right now. You will never be here again. Too much focus on arriving at a destination can lead to a life without joy. Enjoy all the sights you see along the way. Have fun!

Ideal Place

Make sure you have a bright, clutter-free space to practice in. A mirror can provide great feedback on your form and alignment. You can pick up mirrors cheaply at hardware and discount department stores and even more cheaply at glass companies. If you're doing your cross-training away from home, any flat space where you can lie down and move your arms and legs freely will do fine. If you're outside in a park, picnic tables work great as practice space if the ground is wet, uneven, or sloping.

Your Tools

Pilates mats are usually ⅝-inch thick. My favorite is the Balanced Body Aeromat available at www.pilates.com. Yoga mats are usually too thin and make what can be an otherwise enjoyable rolling exercise unpleasant. Two yoga mats stacked work fine, as does a single camping mat. When you go on trips, be sure to toss your mat or camping pad in your car.

You'll also want to get your hands on a stretch band and a set of light-weight dumbbells. I recommend a maximum of two to five pounds. These can be purchased inexpensively at home fitness stores. You can find stretch bands and small dumbbells at discount department stores as well. One- to two-pound ankle weights are also helpful for increasing the intensity of leg exercises, such as Side Kicks.

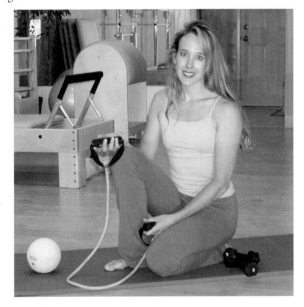

Chapter 6

Rock and Ice Climbers

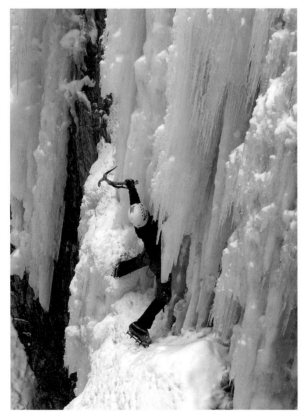

Katie Cahill-Volpe, Ouray Ice Park, Colorado.

As a climber, have you ever wished you were a little taller so you could make a big reach, or a little more flexible for a high step? Have you ever resorted to picking up your foot and placing it where you wanted it to go because you didn't have the flexibility to get there in the first place?

Practicing Pilates, you'll find that monster stems, killer high steps, and sketchy rock-over moves get easier. Likewise, climbing the steepest walls and the blankest slabs requires core strength for body tension. Boost your core strength, and you'll increase your staying power. You'll press harder through your feet, tighten up your line of energy, and take weight off your arms and shoulders.

Dancing over Stone

The best climbers make climbing look like ballet. They are graceful and powerful, flowing from one handhold to the next. A good climber is first and foremost an efficient mover, executing a sequence of movements with precision, control, and flowing motion. Watch Tommy Caldwell and Beth Rodden free-climb El Capitan; their movements are seamless and appear effortless. Achieving this kind of flow requires fitness, skill, and a mind-body connection.

Climbing and Pilates are both movement disciplines that, when done well, are poetry in motion. By practicing Pilates, you'll improve the quality of your fitness and climbing. Not only will you log more pitches in a single day, you'll climb them in better style.

Mental fitness is equally important to a climber. Climbing is dangerous, making even the bravest of us jittery. To climb well and stay safe requires being in control of your mental game. There is no room for distraction or doubt when there is open space between your heels and the ground. Pilates helps you cultivate a strong mind-body connection by improving your awareness, breathing, and focus.

Before diving into the Pilates for Climbers routines, it will benefit you in your quest for fitness and longevity to address the common overuse injuries and training needs of climbers.

Overuse Injuries

One of the major reasons climbers stop climbing is due to overuse injuries. Many climbers overclimb, under-cross-train, and do not take time to fully recover from the stresses of climbing. To make matters worse, many climbers fail to warm up properly before testing their limits or neglect cross-training exercise altogether. Sound like anyone you know? What results are overuse injuries that keep climbers away from the crags and desperate for relief. Following is a list of the most common overuse climbing injuries that could be prevented through proper warm-ups, cross-training, and rest. For more information about these injuries, please refer to Appendix C.

Fingers:
• Finger Pulley Strains and Ruptures
Shoulders:
• Subluxation (Dislocation)
  Impingement
Elbows:
• Lateral Epicondylitis (Tennis Elbow)
• Medial Epicondylitis (Golfer's Elbow)

The higher the grade and the more you climb, the greater the stress load on your body and the more at risk you become for an overuse injury. Preventing overuse injuries means maintaining uniform muscle balance in the forearms, upper arms, and shoulders. Muscle imbalances are responsible for many injuries to the shoulders and elbows. Overly developed back muscles and underdeveloped rotator cuff muscles often lead to shoulder injury. Meanwhile, overdeveloped flexors of the forearms and wrists paired with underdeveloped extensor muscles can lead to elbow injuries. Some of these imbalances may have become apparent in your SWOT self-analysis in Chapter 4.

Maintaining your longevity as a climber means recognizing when you're climbing poorly and choosing to take on the rope or call it a day. Poor form accelerates fatigue, and fatigue begets movement that makes belayers wince. How many times have you seen a climber pumped out of his mind shamelessly making injury-prone movements all for a single climb?

Climbing too much, doing the same moves too many times, and not resting are a formula for disaster. As a general rule, avoid increasing frequency, climbing grade, or volume by more than 10 percent in a given week. Remember: the quality of your training is more important than the quantity. You should only increase one factor at a time in a given week, climb no more than four days a week, and allow at least 48 hours' rest between power workouts to allow adequate rest for muscles and soft tissues to repair. Overuse injuries don't happen in a single cragging day, they cultivate over time. Listen to your body.

7 Tips for Avoiding Injury

1. Warm up on easy climbs and stretch.

2. Maintain uniform muscle balance in your shoulders, arms, and hands.

3. Climb in control and use good technique.

4. While climbing, keep your weight centered over your hips.

5. Avoid climbs beyond your current skills and fitness.

6. Follow the 10 percent rule. Choose to increase your training intensity by 10 percent in one of the following ways in a given week: frequency, climbing grade, or volume. For example, if you increase your climbing days, avoid increasing the grade and number of routes per day.

7. Listen to your body and lay off if you feel pain. If you feel pain, identify its location, what activity seemed to cause it, and monitor any changes. If the pain persists, see a qualified professional before it becomes chronic.

Rock and Ice Climbers

53

THE PILATES PRESCRIPTION: 15 MINUTES A DAY

Creating Balance

An effective Pilates cross-training routine focuses on boosting core strength, improving flexibility, and restoring muscle balance. To begin, let's identify the overused climbing muscles that require stretching and the underused muscles that require strengthening. Please note that some muscles may fall into both categories.

MUSCLES TO STRENGTHEN AND STRETCH

	STRETCH	STRENGTHEN
Upper Body	Latissimus Dorsi	Rotator Cuff
	Upper Trapezius	Pectorals
	Serratus Anterior	Mid-Trapezius
	Back Extensors	Lower Trapezius
	Biceps	Rhomboids
	Triceps	Triceps
	Forearm Flexors	Forearm Extensors
	Wrist Flexors	Wrist Extensors
Core	Hip Flexors	Abdominals
	Hip Extensors	Hip Extensors
	Erector Spinae	Hip Abductors
	Quadratus Lumborum	Hip Adductors
Lower Body	Quadriceps	Shins (Tibialis Anterior)
	Hamstrings	
	Iliotibial Band	
	Calves (Gastronemius and Soleus)	

15-Minute Prescription

The beauty of Pilates exercises is that you can simultaneously stretch one part of your body while strengthening another part. On the following pages are two 15-minute routines. They are designed to meet the cross-training needs of a climber. Alternate between the two routines during your practice three to five times a week. For a complete 30- to 45-minute full-body general-conditioning Pilates workout, refer to the classical routines presented in Part III. For all routines, exercise descriptions are provided in Part III—Your Toolbox. The exercises are ordered in a way that adheres most closely to the Classical Mat Sequence. The sequence is designed to warm up the body and spine and create a satisfying and continuous flow of movement. Use these pages as reference. I encourage you to make a copy for easy use when cross-training at the climbing gym or on a trip.

One Size Doesn't Fit All

Your area of preference, grade of climbing, and frequency are all factors that influence your training needs. While alpine ascents might make your legs the size of logs, steep sport climbs or bouldering might turn your forearms into bricks. No matter what type of climbing you prefer, core strength, flexibility, and uniform muscle development are key. Even if you never leave your local climbing gym, this triad creates a foundation for performing your best and avoiding injury as you pull on crimps, slopers, and side pulls. By no means should you feel compelled to do only the following routines. This book contains more than 80 exercises, enabling you to create a variety of routines to meet your needs. If you choose to design your own routine, use your SWOT analysis in Chapter 4 for guidance and refer to the Pilates Exercise Reference Chart in Appendix A. Use the worksheet in Appendix B to create your own Pilates prescription.

Pilates for Climbers

Goal:
Boost core strength

Uniformly balance muscles

Improve flexibility

Formula:
Strengthen the abdominal and back muscles

Strengthen non-climbing muscles (antagonists)

Stretch climbing muscles (agonists)

Routine A

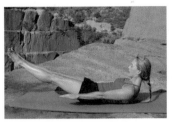

1. The Hundred, page 130

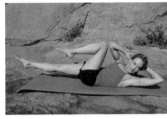

5. Crisscross, page 183

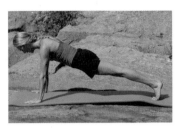

9. Push-Ups, page 168

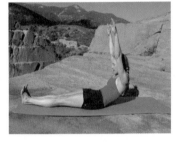

2. Roll Up, page 132

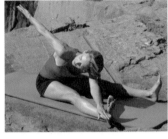

6. Saw, page 145

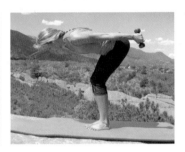

10. Triceps Kickbacks, page 208

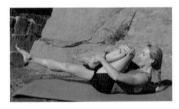

3. One-Leg Stretch, page 139

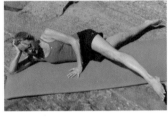

7. Side Kick Series (choose 3–5 variations), pages 171–178

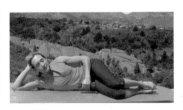

11. Rotator Cuff, page 201

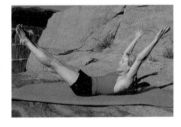

4. Double-Leg Stretch, page 140

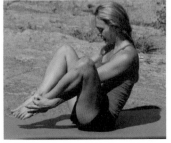

8. Seal, page 166

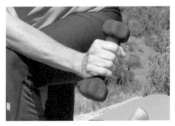

12. Wrist Curls, page 209

Routine B

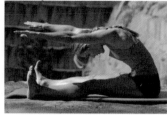

1. Footwork, page 187

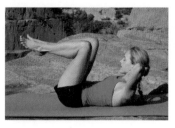

2. Tree, page 193

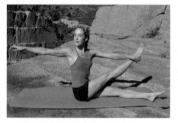

3. Rolling Like a Ball, page 138

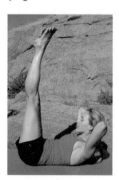

4. Double-Straight-Leg Stretch, page 185

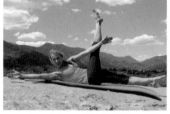

5. Spine Stretch, page 141

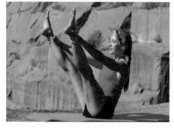

6. Crossover, page 184

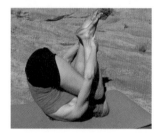

7. Open-Leg Rocker, page 142

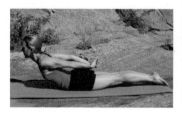

8. Double-Leg Kick, page 148

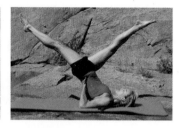

9. Scissors, page 150

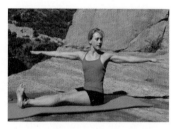

10. Spine Twist, page 153

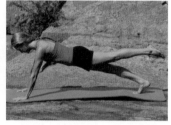

11. Leg Pull-Front, page 160

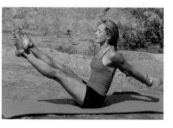

12. Boomerang, page 164

Pilates Boosts

The following section contains Pilates exercises for specific types of climbing. Once you have gained confidence with Routines A and B, add these exercises, if appropriate. You will also find after-climbing stretches and six tips for incorporating Pilates principles into your climbing.

Boosts for Trad Climbing, Ice Climbing, and Big Walling

Trad, ice, and big walling often require long approaches. In addition, steep desert talus, alpine traverses, and endless rope work are often standard fare. They require more strength and endurance in the legs and hips. If you find yourself climbing long routes or your aspirations lead you to alpine settings, add the following exercises to your routine:

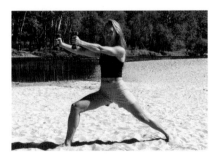

1. Side Lunges, page 179

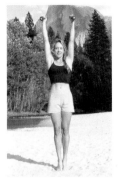

2.
Arm Circles,
page 194

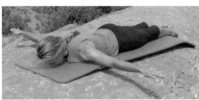

3. T-Bird, page192

Boosts for Sport Climbing and Bouldering

Sport climbing and bouldering use techniques such as heel-hooks and knee-bars, requiring additional strength in the hamstrings, inner thighs, and hips. Boosting core strength makes cross-through moves easier as you twist from your hips instead of your knees. Add these exercises to increase your core strength:

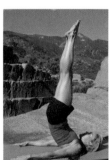

1.
Jackknife,
page 154

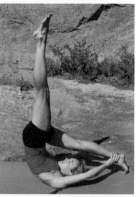

2. Control Balance, page 167

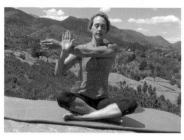

2. Shoulder Stretch, page 218

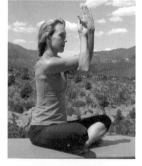

3. Rhomboid Stretch, page 217

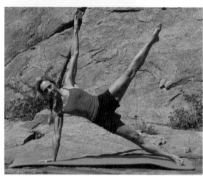

3. Star, page 207

After-Climbing Stretches

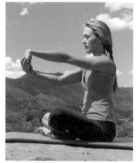

4. Forearm Stretch, page 213

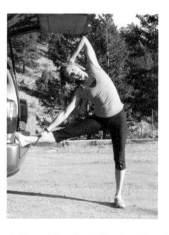

1. Two-Minute Tailgate Stretches, page 218

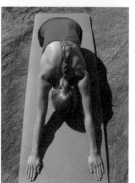

5. Child's Pose, page 212

Pilates in Action:
Six Tips for Climbers

To maximize the integration of Pilates principles from the mat to the crags, here are six exercises to integrate your skills. Choose an easy warm-up that's well below your ability and experiment with each exercise separately. Keep these tips in mind as a checklist for enhancing the efficiency of your training.

1. **Breathing:** Create a rhythm of breathing deeply and coordinate it with your climbing pace. For example, inhale to pause before a move, exhale deeply as you commit to a move.

2. **Centering:** Engage your core. When executing powerful moves such as deadpoints or dynos, pull your navel to your spine. Try this on moves requiring increased body tension, such as on steep overhangs or friction slabs. Stay centered in your core and coordinate the movement of your limbs around your center of gravity.

3. **Concentration:** Strengthen your mind-body connection. Practice climbing in a style that is focused on solving the task at hand. For example, if you are working a red-point that's currently at your limit, focus your attention on making clips from optimal stances and maximizing rests.

4. **Control:** Calculate the amount of power and strength required for each movement. Where appropriate, experiment with static and dynamic movement that is in control.

5. **Fluid Motion:** Transition seamlessly from one move to the next. Allow your movement to be fluid and rhythmic. Practice this skill while doing rock-overs, stems, and delicate slab moves.

6. **Precision:** Watch your feet. Place and weight them with precision. Practice precision with handholds as well. Decide on a precise grip and arm position.

Chapter 7

Road Cyclists and Mountain Bikers

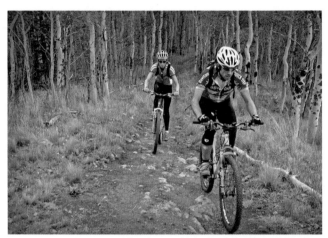

Posture, pedal cadence, and technical skill make the elite rider shine. Whether you are riding a century or tackling mountain-biking obstacles, physical and mental fitness contribute to better balance, agility, and handling skills. To maintain a low aerodynamic position and maximize pedaling efficiency, a rider must possess core strength, flexibility, and good alignment. Technical skills such as standing, sprinting, and hopping require upper-body strength. Dealing with obstacles and persevering when the going gets tough require mental fortitude. Improving your mind-body connection begins with improving your breathing.

Road cycling and mountain biking utilize the same major muscle groups yet build fitness slightly differently. Road cycling builds fitness by maintaining constant cruising speeds over long periods of time, whereas mountain biking builds fitness by placing variable demands on a cyclist's energy and power. The cross-training needs of the two vary in that a mountain biker requires more upper-body strength, agility, and balance, while a road biker requires leg strength, cardiovascular fitness, and pedal technique. By participating in both types of riding, you can further improve your overall fitness and riding skills.

Whether you're a roadie, dirt lovin' mountain biker, or recreational cyclist, Pilates will help you ride smoother, pedal longer, and avoid injury. While cycling improves cardiovascular fitness and lower-body endurance, Pilates boosts core strength, flexibility, and muscle balance. Core strength is essential to maintaining a still torso while the legs generate force by peddling. If your core is weak, the force generated by your legs will be absorbed into your back. A strong core is key to achieving pedaling power and efficiency. By stretching your upper body, you will gain greater range of motion and health in your shoulders, arms, and torso. By improving flexibility and muscle balance, you'll minimize energy expenditure, be less prone to injury, and experience a more comfortable ride.

Before diving into the Pilates for Cyclists routines, familiarizing yourself with common overuse injuries and the training needs of cyclists will serve you in your quest to perform your best and enjoy many more rides.

Overuse Injuries

The harder you ride, the more at risk you become for an overuse injury. The following is a list of the most common riding injuries. For more information about these injuries, please refer to Appendix C.

Feet:
• Achilles Tendonitis
Knees:
• Chondromalacia
• Patellofemoral Pain Syndrome (Runner's Knee)
• Patella Tendonitis (Jumper's Knee)
• Plica Syndrome

Legs:
• Iliotibial-Band Syndrome
• Biceps Femoris Tendonitis
Neck:
• Shermer's Neck
Hand and Wrist:
• Carpal Tunnel Syndrome
• De Quervains Disease (DQD)
• Ulnar Neuritis (Biker's Wrist)

Most cycling injuries affect the knees. Pedaling is a repetitive and labor-intensive motion that creates muscular imbalances in the legs and hips, stressing the soft tissues of the knee. The average cadence of a road cyclist is 90 revolutions per minute. That equates to 5,400 strokes per hour. This is a faster cadence than in mountain biking, but it is also steadier. Mountain bikers change their pedal cadence continuously as they adapt to changing terrain, often requiring them to shift up to 100 times per hour. For this reason, road cyclists tend to experience more injury to the knees and mountain bikers tend to experience more injury to the hands and thumbs.

Muscle Imbalances

Muscle imbalances are created from the front to the back and from the right to left leg if one leg is favored more on the downstroke. Pedal power is derived from the quadriceps and hip extensors. Although cycling uses the hamstrings continuously, the quadriceps muscles dominate. Therefore, additional hamstring strength is required to bring the legs into balance. Structural misalignments can also create imbalance. Riders with leg-length discrepancy, wider hips, or "knock-knees" are more at risk for developing knee injuries due to the higher probability of kneecap misalignment. Pilates helps improve alignment by improving posture, muscle balance, and awareness. Leg stability and alignment are improved by strengthening the abductors (outer thighs) and adductors (inner thighs). Balanced muscles that are flexible and strong improve alignment, alleviate muscular tension on the knees, and reduce the risk of injury.

Training Mistakes

Training mistakes such as riding too many miles too quickly, pushing too big of a gear, and inadequate warm-ups are a formula for injury. As is true with other sports, avoid increasing frequency, intensity, or mileage by more than 10 percent in a given week, and only increase one factor at a time in a given week.

Misfits

You could do everything right, but if your bike doesn't fit, your risk of injury is magnified. Improper frame size, saddle height, crank length, stem dimensions, cleat position, and handlebar angle have been known to cause injury. A saddle that is too high causes excessive hip motion while pedaling, whereas a saddle that is too low causes excessive knee bending and loss of power. If you plan to log some miles, it is best to get a professional bike fit.

7 Tips for Avoiding Injury

1. Warm up before pushing yourself, and remember to stretch after your ride.
2. Maintain uniform muscle balance in your hips, legs, and feet.
3. Maintain flexibility, strength, and range of motion in your torso and upper body.
4. While riding, engage your core and stabilize your torso.
5. Maintain good form and technique.
6. Follow the 10 percent rule. Choose to increase only one of the following three factors by 10 percent in a given week: intensity, frequency, or volume.
7. Listen to your body. If you feel pain, identify its location, what activity caused it, and monitor changes. If the pain persists, see a qualified professional before it becomes chronic.

Creating Balance

An effective Pilates cross-training routine focuses on boosting core strength, improving flexibility, and restoring muscle balance. To begin, let's identify the overused cycling muscles that require stretching and the underused muscles that require strengthening. Please note that some muscles may fall into both categories.

CYCLING MUSCLES TO STRETCH AND STRENGTHEN

	STRETCH	STRENGTHEN
Lower Body	Quadriceps	Hamstrings
	Hamstrings	
	Iliotibial Band	
	Shins (Tibialis Anterior)	
	Calves (Gastronemius and Soleus)	
Core	Hip Flexors	Abdominals
	Hip Extensors	Hip Abductors
	Hip Adductors	Quadratus Lumborum
		Erector Spinae
Upper Body	Latissimus Dorsi	Latissimus Dorsi
	Pectorals	Pectorals
	Serratus Anterior	Rhomboids
	Neck Extensors	Neck Flexors
	Mid Trapezius	
	Upper Trapezius	Lower Trapezius
	Forearm Flexors	Forearm Extensors
	Wrist Flexors	Wrist Extensors
	Biceps and Triceps	Biceps and Triceps

15-Minute Pilates Prescription

The beauty of Pilates exercises is that you can simultaneously stretch one part of your body while strengthening another part. On the following pages are two 15-minute routines. They are designed to meet the cross-training needs of a cyclist. Alternate between the two routines during your practice three to five times a week. For a complete 30- to 45-minute full-body general-conditioning Pilates workout, refer to the classical routines presented in Part III. For all routines, exercise descriptions are provided in Part III: Your Toolbox. The exercises are ordered in a way that adheres most closely to the Classical Mat Sequence. The sequence is designed to warm up the body and spine and create a satisfying and continuous flow of movement. Use these pages as a reference. I encourage you to make a copy for easy use when cross-training at the gym or on a trip.

One Size Doesn't Fit All

The type of riding you do, including its difficulty, duration, and frequency, will influence your training needs. While road cycling requires lower-body and cardiovascular endurance, mountain biking also requires upper-body strength. No matter what type of riding you prefer, core strength, flexibility, and uniform muscle development are key. This triad creates a foundation for performing your best and avoiding injury. By no means should you feel compelled to do only the following routines. This book contains more than 80 exercises, enabling you to create a variety of routines to suit your needs. If you choose to design your own routine, use your SWOT self-analysis from Chapter 4 for guidance and refer to the Pilates Exercise Reference Chart in Appendix A. Use the worksheet in Appendix B to create your own Pilates prescription.

Pilates for Cyclists

Goal:

Boost core strength

Uniformly balance muscles

Improve flexibility

Formula:

Strengthen the abdominal and back muscles

Strengthen non-cycling muscles (antagonists)

Stretch cycling muscles (agonists)

Routine A

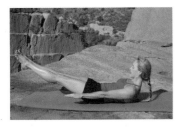

1. The Hundred, page 130

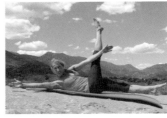

5. Crisscross, page 183

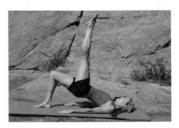

9. Shoulder Bridge with Kicks, page 152

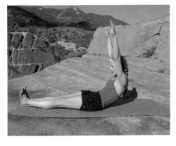

2. Roll Up, page 132

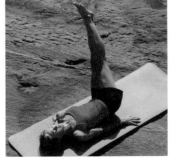

6. Corkscrew, page 144

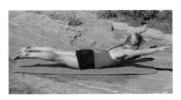

10. Swimming or Skydiver, page 159 or 189

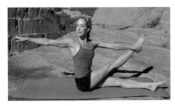

3. Tree, page 193

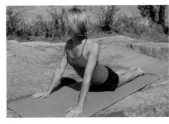

7. Neck Roll, page 216

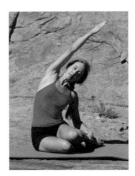

11. Mermaid, page 215

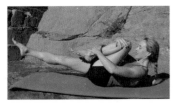

4. One-Leg Stretch, page 139

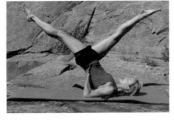

8. Scissors, page 150

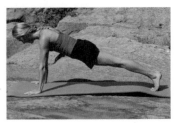

12. Push-Ups, page 168

Routine B

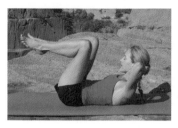

1. Footwork, page 187

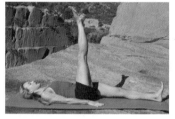

2. One-Leg Circles, page 136

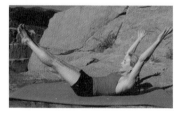

3. Double-Leg Stretch, page 140

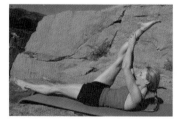

4. One-Straight-Leg Stretch, page 188

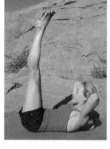

5. Double-Straight-Leg Stretch, page 185

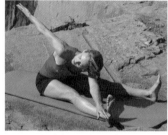

6. Saw, page 145

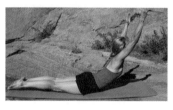

7. Swan Dive, page 146

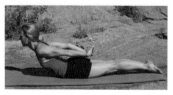

8. Double-Leg Kick, page 148

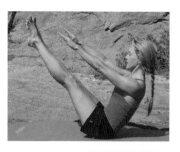

9. Teaser Series, page 156

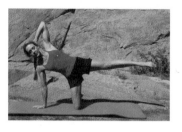

10. Kneeling Side Kicks, page 162

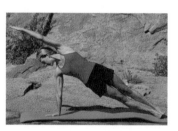

11. Side Bend, page 163

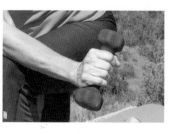

12. Wrist Curls, page 209

Road Cyclists and Mountain Bikers

THE PILATES PRESCRIPTION: 15 MINUTES A DAY

Pilates Boosts

The following section contains Pilates exercises for specific types of riding. Once you have gained confidence with Routines A and B, add these exercises, if appropriate. In this section, you will also find after-riding stretches and six tips for incorporating Pilates principles into your biking.

Boosts for Road Cyclists

Road cyclists benefit from additional lower-body endurance and core strength.

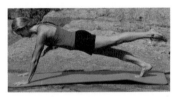

1. Leg Pull-Front, page 160

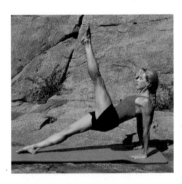

2. Leg Pull-Up, page 161

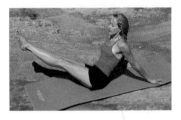

3. Hip Circles, page 158

Boosts for Mountain Bikers

Mountain bikers benefit from additional upper-body strength, agility, and balance for bunny hops, tight corners, and steep hills. To simultaneously boost upper-body and core strength, add the following exercises to your cross-training routine:

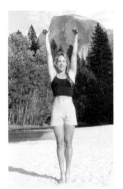

1. Arm Circles, page 194

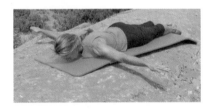

2. T-Bird, page 192

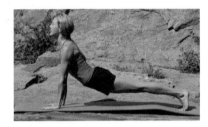

3. Snake, page 190

Boosts for Recumbent Riders

Recumbent bikes mean more surface of your rump on the saddle. This creates additional tightness for the hip extensor and flexor muscles. To stretch these muscles, add the following exercises to your cross-training routine:

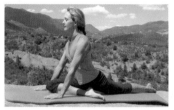

1. Pigeon Pose, page 216

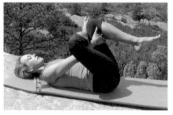

2. Figure 4, page 212

After-Riding Stretches

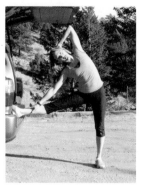

1. Two-Minute Tailgate Stretches, page 218

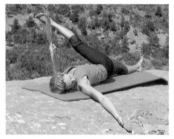

2. Leg Stretch with Band, page 214

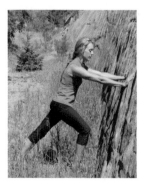

3. Calves Stretch, page 211

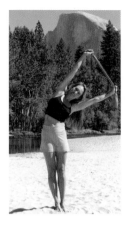

4. Upper-Body Band Stretches, page 219

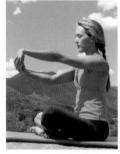

5. Forearm Stretch, page 213

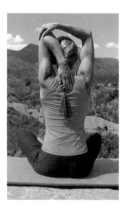

6. Triceps Stretch, page 219

Road Cyclists and Mountain Bikers

69

THE PILATES PRESCRIPTION: 15 MINUTES A DAY

Pilates in Action:
Six Tips for Cyclists

To maximize the integration of Pilates from the mat to the bike, apply these six principles while pedaling. Experiment with each one separately on your next ride and keep them in mind as a checklist for enhancing the efficiency of your cadence.

1. **Breathing:** Breathing deeply and establishing a rhythm that paces well with your cadence improves muscular endurance and helps you stay focused even in the most challenging conditions. Create a rhythm of breathing and coordinate it with your cycling stroke. Once you've been successful maintaining a pattern, experiment with new ones.

2. **Centering:** Engage your core. Keep your back flat like a tabletop and draw your navel to your spine. You could also pretend that your bike shorts have a zipper holding your abdomen in firmly. By keeping your torso still and minimizing energy lost in rocking back and forth, you place more energy into pedaling.

3. **Concentration:** Strengthen your mind-body connection. Practice riding in a style that is present and focused on the task at hand. Focus on keeping your torso still, your shoulders relaxed, and your pedal stroke round and consistent.

4. **Control:** Use control to create consistent and smooth pedaling and minimize torso movement. A cadence monitor is a great way to keep your revolutions per minute up and to monitor your efficiency. In general, uphill cadences tend to be lower than downhill, unless you are Lance Armstrong and maintain a very high cadence even on steep inclines.

5. **Fluid Motion:** As you pedal, create a circle of flowing motion that is seamless. Feel the roundness of each stroke and create a sense of continuous effort on the downstroke and upstroke so there is no beginning or end. You'll engage your legs more evenly and reduce fatigue.

6. **Precision:** Be precise. Be more concerned about maintaining the best possible form than about speed. Be quiet and still in your torso, relaxed in the shoulders, elbows, and jaw, and avoid overgripping the handlebars. By doing so you have a better chance of avoiding injury and numbness and improving efficiency. Keep your body centered over your bike minimizing movement while you pedal. The more still your torso, the more precise your pedaling.

Chapter 8

Hikers, Backpackers, and Snowshoers

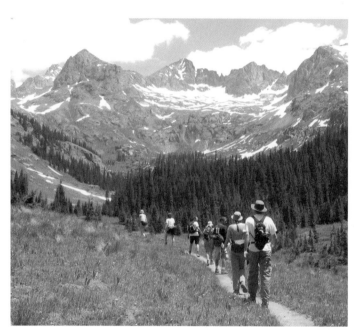

Whether your journey takes you through oak forests, aspen groves, or alpine slopes, hiking, snowshoeing, and backpacking encourage you to slow down, open your eyes, examine your surroundings, and take your time. Going by foot offers an opportunity to be present, reconnect with the earth, and also reconnect with yourself. If you want to make the least impact on your knees, hips, and back, you've chosen the right outdoor activity. And if you are looking to lose weight, snowshoeing burns as many calories as running, without the impact. Whether you go by foot or snowshoe, for a day trip or many nights, Pilates is the perfect complement to your cardiovascular fitness training.

Walking Tall

Most people take about 2,000 steps for every mile they walk. The average walker steps about 8,000 times per hour. The quality of your gait influences the wear and tear on your joints. While striding, many people tend to lead with one leg. This can result in muscle imbalances not only from front to back but also from left to right. In addition, striding longer with one leg than the other creates imbalances.

Improving the quality of your gait can mean the difference between pleasure and pain. A good gait minimizes energy expenditure, reduces impact on your back and knees, and creates a more comfortable outing. Pilates can help you improve your gait by improving your posture, breathing, core strength, and muscle balance.

Standing up tall and aligning your body improves joint range of motion, takes pressure off your back, and improves your breathing. A strong core helps you to stay light and lifted over your feet. Boosting your core strength also improves your balance and agility so the next time you cross a river, hop a boulder field, or traverse a snowy slope, you'll have more confidence. To walk a steady pace for many miles requires breathing deeply to provide your muscles with oxygen-rich blood. Proper breathing improves muscular endurance, enabling you to tackle the most challenging terrain. By inhaling through the nose and exhaling through the mouth, you'll stay tuned in to your heart rate and exertion levels, dehydrate less quickly, and, because nose breathing stimulates the parasympathetic nervous system, you'll feel calmer. Maintaining

muscle balance in the lower body is also important for posture and alignment.

Balanced muscles that are flexible and strong enhance gait and reduce the risk of injury. Additional strength and flexibility in your legs and hips take pressure off your knees, improve range of motion, and also improve your endurance. If you're carrying a pack or poling, boosting upper-body strength is also beneficial. Pilates can help you improve your gait by improving your alignment, core strength, and overall fitness. Before diving into the Pilates for Walkers routines, it will benefit you to address the most common overuse injuries and muscle-balance needs of the walking enthusiast.

Overuse Injuries

The following is a list of the most common hiking, backpacking, and snowshoeing injuries.

Feet:
• Blisters
• Plantar Fasciitis
Knees:
• Chondromalacia Patellofemoral
  Pain Syndrome (Runner's Knee)
• Patella Tendonitis (Jumper's Knee)
• Plica Syndrome
Legs:
• Iliotibial-Band Syndrome

Overuse injuries can be caused by a number of things, including improper footwear, poor posture and gait, lack of proper fitness, and training mistakes.

Misfits

Something as small as a blister can ruin an outing. Wearing crummy shoes or a poor-fitting backpack can lead to injury. Replacing footwear on a timely basis is important. Backpacks should be properly fitted to your body. Make sure the pack's position doesn't compromise the alignment of your neck and back and that the weight is centered on your hips. Your pack should be stable and not shift side to side when you bend and turn.

Misalignments

Structural misalignments in your body can affect the quality of your gait. Foot misalignment can lead to ankle, knee, hip, and back injuries. Leg length discrepancy creates imbalanced work between each leg and can cause injury. Walkers with wider hips or with higher Q-angles (the quadriceps angle is measured by a line drawn from the front side of your hip bone [the anterior superior iliac spine] to the center of your kneecap, and another line drawn from the center of your kneecap to just below where the patellar tendon inserts) or who are "knock-kneed" are more at risk for injuries due to misalignment. Many structural misalignments can

be corrected by improving your gait, muscle balance, and by using proper footwear and arch supports.

Imbalances

Muscle imbalances such as overly tight hamstrings, calves, and hips and underdeveloped vastus medialis obliques (VMO) interfere with proper alignment and create excess muscle tension between the kneecap and upper leg bone, which often leads to knee injuries. By uniformly strengthening and stretching the muscles of your legs and hips, you'll reduce your risk of injury as you walk terrain that slopes and changes with every step.

Excesses

Adding too many miles too fast is a formula for injury. The repetitive motion of striding is demanding on the soft tissues of the knees. Mistakes such as not stretching, increasing distances and terrain difficulty too quickly, and overexertion have consequences. An extended backpacking trip that does not allow the body adequate recovery time can contribute to overuse injuries of the knee.

7 Tips for Avoiding Injury

1. Warm up, and remember to stretch.

2. Maintain uniform muscle balance in your hips, legs, and feet.

3. Avoid walks beyond your current fitness level.

4. While walking, engage your core for support.

5. Maintain good posture and gait.

6. Follow the 10 percent rule. Choose to increase only one of the following factors by 10 percent in a given week: intensity, frequency, or volume.

7. Listen to your body. If you feel pain, identify its location, what activity seemed to cause it, and monitor any changes. If the pain persists, see a qualified professional before it becomes chronic.

Creating Balance

Hiking, backpacking, and snowshoeing are energy-absorbing aerobic sports that require lower-body strength and endurance. An effective Pilates cross-training routine focuses on boosting core strength, improving flexibility, and restoring muscle balance. To begin, let's identify the primary muscles that require stretching and the muscles that require strengthening. Please note that some muscles may fall into both categories.

MUSCLES TO STRETCH AND STRENGTHEN

	STRETCH	STRENGTHEN
Lower Body	Quadriceps	Medial Quadriceps
	Hamstrings	Hamstrings
	Iliotibial Band	Shins (Tibialis Anterior)
	Calves (Gastronemius and Soleus)	
Core	Hip Flexors	Abdominals
	Hip Extensors	Hip Abductors
	Hip Adductors	
Upper Body	Upper Trapezius	Lower and Mid-Trapezius
		Pectorals

15-Minute Pilates Prescription

The beauty of Pilates exercises is that you can simultaneously stretch one part of your body while strengthening another part. On the following pages are two 15-minute routines. They are designed to meet the cross-training needs of a walker. Alternate between the two routines during your practice three to five times a week. For a complete 30- to 45-minute full-body general-conditioning Pilates workout, refer to the classical routines presented in Part III. For all routines, exercise descriptions are provided in Part III: Your Toolbox. The exercises are ordered in a way that adheres most closely to the Classical Mat Sequence. The sequence is designed to warm up the body and spine and create a satisfying and continuous flow of movement. Use these pages as a reference. I encourage you to make a copy for easy use when cross-training at the gym or on a trip.

One Size Doesn't Fit All

The type of walking you do and its difficulty, duration, and frequency determine your training needs. While day hikes and snowshoeing will tone your legs, backpacking may build muscle mass in your lower and upper body. No matter what type of walking you prefer, core strength, flexibility, and uniform muscle development are key. This triad creates a foundation for performing your best and avoiding injury. By no means should you feel compelled to do only the following routines. This book contains more than 80 exercises, enabling you to create a variety of routines to meet your needs. If you choose to design your own routine, use your SWOT self-analysis from Chapter 4 for guidance and refer to the Pilates Exercise Reference Chart in Appendix A. Use the worksheet in Appendix B to create your own Pilates prescription.

Pilates for Walkers

Goal:

Boost core strength

Uniformly balance muscles

Improve flexibility

Formula:

Strengthen the abdominal and back muscles

Strengthen non-walking muscles (antagonists)

Stretch walking muscles (agonists)

Routine A

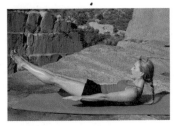

1. The Hundred, page 130

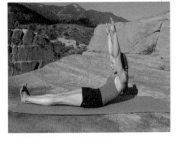

2. Roll Up, page 132

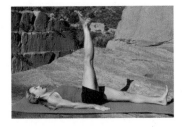

3. One-Leg Circles, page 136

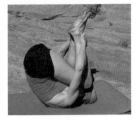

4. Rolling Like a Ball, page 138

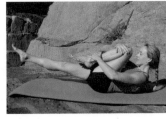

5. One-Leg Stretch, page 139

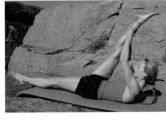

6. One-Straight-Leg Stretch, page 188

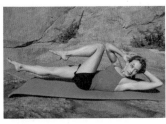

7. Crisscross, page 183

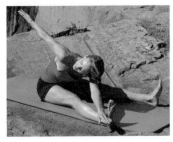

8. Saw, page 145

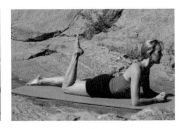

9. One-Leg Kick, page 147

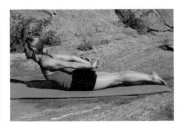

10. Double-Leg Kick, page 148

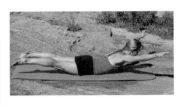

11. Swimming or Skydiver, page 159 or 189

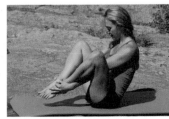

12. Seal, page 166

Routine B

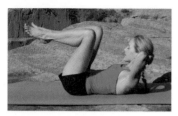

1. Footwork, page 187

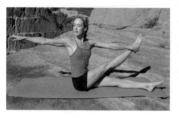

2. Tree, page 193

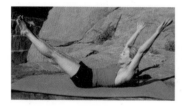

3. Double-Leg Stretch, page 140

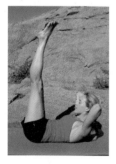

4. Double-Straight-Leg Stretch, page 185

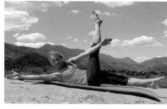

5. Crossover, page 184

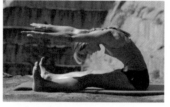

6. Spine Stretch, page 141

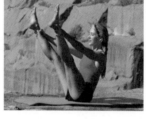

7. Open-Leg Rocker, page 142

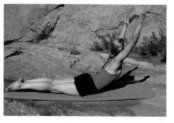

8. Swan Dive or Swan Rocking, page 146 or 191

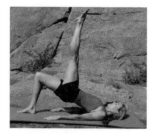

9. Shoulder Bridge with Kicks, page 152

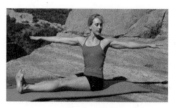

10. Spine Twist, page 153

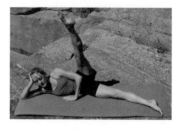

11. Side Kicks Series (choose 3–5), pages 171–178

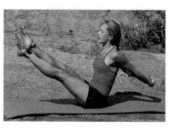

12. Boomerang, page 164

Pilates Boosts

To boost your training, combine the leg and hip exercises from Routines A and B into a single session or add one of the full-body conditioning Pilates routines in Part III to your weekly practice. The following section contains Pilates exercises for specific types of walking. In this section, you will also find after-walking stretches and six tips for incorporating Pilates principles into your treks.

Boosts for Backpackers

Whether you aspire to experience all 211 miles of the John Muir Trail or a weekend exploring Utah's labyrinthine canyons, Pilates cross-training is a great complement to your cardiovascular training. Living in untouched wilderness and being self-sufficient requires both physical and mental fitness. Backpackers benefit from additional upper-body strength, leg strength, and balance to lift and carry a pack without strain. To simultaneously boost upper-body and core strength, add the following exercises to your cross-training routine:

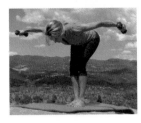

1. Bug, page 195

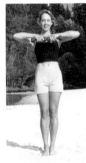

2. Zip-Ups, page 210

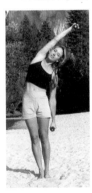

3. Side-to-Side, page 205

Boosts for Walkers with Poles

Adding poles to your walking creates a full-body workout. Poling strengthens the muscles of your arms, shoulders, and back. It also improves cardiovascular fitness and adds power and speed to your walking. When tackling steep and rocky terrain or carrying a backpack, poles help reduce impact on the knees and improve balance. Athletes with knee injuries will find poles useful for minimizing impact. Invest in good poles designed to absorb vibration and shock, otherwise your elbows will. Make certain that the poles can be adjusted to your height, have comfortable ergonomic handgrips, and absorb shock with a spring or a rubber tip. To condition your arms and shoulders for poling, add the following exercises to your routine:

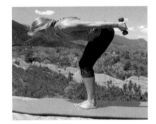

1. Triceps Kickbacks, page 208

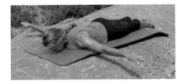

2. T-Bird, page 192

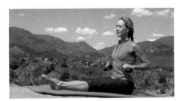

3. Rowing, page 198

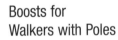

Boosts for Snowshoers

Snowshoeing is a cardio work-out on par with running, making it fabulous off-season training—without the additional stress that running puts on your knees. It is also great for people recovering from knee injuries. Snowshoeing challenges balance more than hiking does and requires additional ankle strength to adapt to changing snow surfaces. Snowshoeing requires endurance and strength. Whether you snowshoe for alpine ascents or for fun and exercise in the winter, you'll experience the benefits of Pilates as you climb and descend slopes.

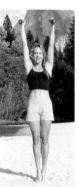

1. Arm Circles, page 194

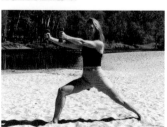

2. Side Lunges, page 179

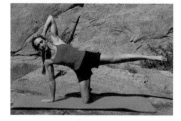

3. Kneeling Side Kicks, page 162

After-Walking Stretches

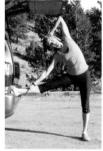

1. Two-Minute Tailgate Stretches, page 218

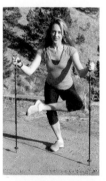

2. Figure 4 with Ski Poles or Hiking Poles, page 213

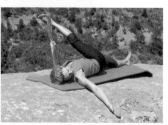

3. Leg Stretch with Band, page 214

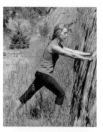

4. Calves Stretch, page 211

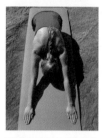

5. Child's Pose, page 212

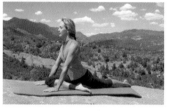

6. Pigeon Pose, page 216

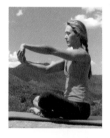

7. Forearm Stretch (for walkers using poles), page 213

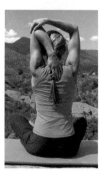

8. Triceps Stretch (for walkers using poles), page 219

Pilates in Action:
Six Tips for Walkers

To maximize the integration of Pilates principles from the mat to the trail, here are six exercises designed to integrate your skills and increase the quality of your gait. Experiment with them on your next outing and keep them in mind to enhance the efficiency of your movement.

1. **Breathing:** Breathe deeply. Create a rhythm of breathing and coordinate it with your walking pace. Set a pace that allows you to breathe freely and comfortably. Practice inhaling deeply and exhaling air completely, drawing your core in tightly.

2. **Centering:** Engage your core by drawing your navel to your spine while you walk. This will give your lower back additional support and center your movements from your core.

3. **Concentration:** Strengthen your mind-body connection. Use your breath and intention to keep you centered and present. Create a gait that maintains good posture and alignment. You will save energy, reduce wear and tear on your joints, and become more present in the moment.

4. **Control:** Avoid using momentum to carry you forward. Keep your movements in control. You'll work your legs more uniformly instead of throwing your legs forward. Stay centered over your hips and minimize up-and-down and side-to-side motion.

5. **Flowing Motion:** Transition seamlessly from one step to the next. Allow your movement to be fluid and rhythmic, carrying you forward like a flowing river.

6. **Precision:** Be precise as you step with your feet and plant with your poles. Precise movement is energy efficient, reduces fatigue and muscle imbalances, and keeps you more solid on uneven terrain.

Chapter 9

Paddlers

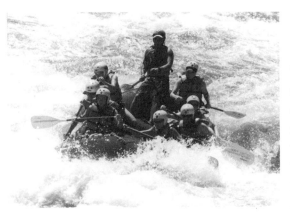

There is something elusive and compelling about water, whether it's a serpentine river, a mountain lake, or the open sea. Like friends, each has its own personality, and we seek them for different reasons. Some water flows calmly and gently, like a whisper. Other water carves out the landscape like a sculptor with clay.

The best paddlers move like the water itself, seamlessly connecting one stroke to the next. Paddling requires a powerful upper body, an equally strong core, and lower-body fitness. The average paddler makes approximately 25 strokes per minute. That equates to 400 strokes per mile and 1,500 per hour. Sea kayaking is even more demanding, with approximately 1,000 strokes per mile, or 3,000 strokes per hour. Whether you kayak or canoe, good posture, core strength, and flexible, balanced muscles are key.

Posture determines the quality of your paddling technique. By stacking your hips, shoulders, and head as if you were sitting against a wall, you improve torso and shoulder range of motion, enable your spine to rotate freely, and allow your lungs to expand fully. Maintaining proper alignment reduces upper-body fatigue, alleviates pressure on your lower back, and reduces risk of injury. Core strength, flexibility, and awareness are the building blocks of good posture. While core strength provides support for the spine, flexibility in the hips and legs enables paddlers to avoid slumping while seated for several hours at a time.

Freedom to Be Fluid

Core strength is the engine that drives torso rotation and other paddling movements. Strong abdominal, hip, and lower-back muscles enable paddlers to generate a dynamic line of energy from the lower body to the upper body, reducing strain on the shoulders and arms and improving everything from hip snaps to Eskimo rolls. Core strength enables paddlers to more effectively tilt a boat and maintain their center of balance. Equally important is flexibility. The more you paddle, the tighter your muscles. Additional flexibility reduces strain in the torso and shoulders and frees the body to twist and adapt to sudden changes along the way.

By adding Pilates to your cross-training, you'll increase your freedom of movement and experience better agility, balance, and reduced risk of injury. Before diving into the Pilates for Paddlers routines, we'll address common overuse injuries and the training needs of paddlers to serve you in your quest to perform your best and enjoy many more outings.

Overuse Injuries

Improving your fitness and paddling technique is the best defense against injury. The most common paddling injuries affect the shoulders, elbows, and wrists.

Shoulders:
• Impingement
• Dislocation (Subluxation)
Elbows:
• Lateral Epicondylitis (Tennis Elbow)
• Medial Epicondylitis (Golfer's Elbow)
Wrists:
• Ulnar Nerve Entrapment
• Carpal Tunnel Syndrome

The more you paddle, the more at risk you become for an overuse injury. Improperly fitted equipment, poor form, and insufficient muscle balance are responsible for many overuse injuries.

Misfits

A kayak that is improperly fitted and paddles that are too heavy create unnecessary stress. A deck that is too low doesn't allow the knees to bend or raise and creates lower-back and leg pain. If your legs are too far apart, they create extra work for your hips. If your feet are unable to press firmly into the footrest, you will brace with your thighs, resulting in muscle cramping, reduced circulation, and less-efficient paddling.

Poor Form

The quality of your posture, technique, and fitness determines the wear and tear on your joints. Paddlers with poor posture increase stress and fatigue in the back, shoulders, and neck and reduce range of motion in the torso. Paddlers with insufficient core strength use their arms to power a stroke instead of their torso and often end up with shoulder injuries. Inadequate abdominal strength causes excessive rounding and arching of the low back, which creates stress on the lumbar spine. Poor technique also creates injury to the wrist and elbow. Excessive cocking of the wrist and overgripping the paddle can create tendonitis in the elbow.

Inadequate Cross-Training

As in other sports, paddling strengthens some muscles as others become weaker. A forward paddle stroke creates back muscles that are stronger than the muscles of the chest. Creating muscle balance requires additional strengthening and stretching of the upper body. Imbalances also occur from left to right. This is common in white-water canoeing as well as with kayakers who have a tendency to pull harder with one arm than the other. Strengthening the muscles of the mid-back and torso adds stability and prevents the upper-back muscles from working excessively, thereby increasing stress on the neck and shoulders.

Paddling requires a wide range of shoulder motion. Repeatedly lifting a paddle all day results in fatigued shoulders and a tight lower back, hips, and legs. Reaching the arms as you power a stroke tightens the muscles in the chest and back. If the water is rough or presents obstacles, tremendous force is placed on the shoulder joint. Balancing the muscles around the shoulder—the rotator cuff muscles, serratus anterior, and pectorals—will help keep the shoulder joint in place and reduce the risk of dislocation or tendonitis. Practicing Pilates exercises will help you to gain the strength, stamina, and awareness to maintain good posture and better paddling technique.

7 Tips for Avoiding Injury

1. Warm up and stretch.

2. Maintain good posture.

3. Avoid paddling beyond your current skills and fitness.

4. While paddling, rotate your torso to create power and finesse.

5. Follow the 10 percent rule. Avoid increasing intensity, frequency, or volume by more than 10 percent in a given week.

6. Maintain muscle balance in your shoulders, back, chest, and arms.

7. Listen to your body and lay off when you feel aches and pains.

Paddlers

83

THE PILATES PRESCRIPTION: 15 MINUTES A DAY

Creating Balance

An effective Pilates cross-training routine focuses on boosting core strength, improving flexibility, and restoring muscle balance. It's important to stretch the overworked paddling muscles and strengthen the underworked non-paddling muscles.

Please note that some muscles may fall into both categories. No matter what paddling activity you do, all rely heavily on core strength to stabilize your boat and transfer power from the lower body to the upper body while paddling.

MUSCLES TO STRETCH AND STRENGTHEN

	STRETCH	STRENGTHEN
Upper Body	Deltoids	Rotator Cuff
	Pectorals	Rhomboids
	Latissimus Dorsi	Pectorals
	Back Extensors	Serratus Anterior
	Upper Trapezius	Mid-Trapezius
	Biceps	Low Trapezius
	Triceps	Triceps
	Forearm Flexors	Forearm Extensors
	Wrist Flexors	Wrist Extensors
Core		Abdominals
	Quadratus Lumborum	Hip Adductors
	Hip Flexors	Hip Abductors
	Hip Extensors	Hip Extensors
Lower Body	Hamstrings	Quadriceps
	Iliotibial Band	
	Calves (Gastronemius and Soleus)	

15-Minute Pilates Prescription

The beauty of Pilates exercises is that you can simultaneously stretch one part of your body while strengthening another part. On the following pages are two 15-minute routines. They are designed to meet the cross-training needs of a paddler. Alternate between the two routines during your practice three to five times a week. For a complete 30- to 45-minute full-body general-conditioning Pilates workout, refer to the classical routines presented in Part III. For all routines, exercise descriptions are provided in Part III: Your Toolbox. The exercises are ordered in a way that adheres most closely to the Classical Mat Sequence. The sequence is designed to warm up the body and spine and create a satisfying and continuous flow of movement. Use these pages as a reference. I encourage you to make a copy for easy use when cross-training at the gym or on a trip.

One Size Doesn't Fit All

The type of paddling you prefer, level of difficulty, and frequency determine your training needs. However, all require core strength, flexibility, and uniform muscle development. This triad creates a foundation for performing your best and avoiding injury. Because your needs may vary, refer to the additional exercises that follow the prescriptions. By no means should you feel compelled to do only the following routines. This book contains more than 80 exercises, enabling you to create a variety of routines to meet your needs. If you choose to design your own routine, use your SWOT self-analysis from Chapter 4 for guidance and refer to the Pilates Exercise Reference Chart in Appendix A. Use the worksheet in Appendix B to create your own Pilates prescription.

Pilates for Paddlers

Goal:

Boost core strength

Uniformly balance muscles

Improve flexibility

Formula:

Strengthen the abdominal and back muscles

Strengthen non-paddling muscles (antagonists)

Stretch paddling muscles (agonists)

Routine A

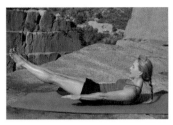

1. The Hundred, page 130

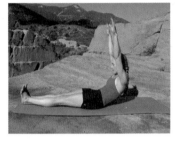

2. Roll Up, page 132

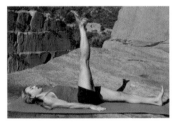

3. One-Leg Circles, page 136

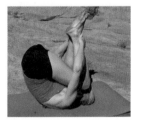

4. Rolling Like a Ball, page 138

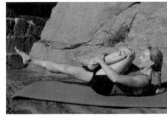

5. One-Leg Stretch, page 139

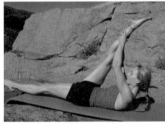

6. One-Straight-Leg Stretch, page 188

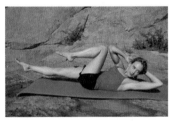

7. Crisscross, page 183

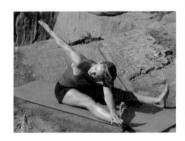

8. Saw, page 145

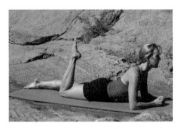

9. One-Leg Kick, page 147

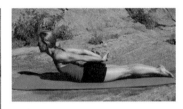

10. Double-Leg Kick, page 148

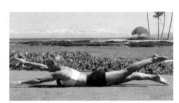

11. Swimming or Skydiver, page 159 or 189

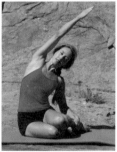

12. Mermaid, page 215

Routine B

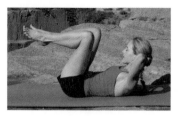

1. Footwork, page 187

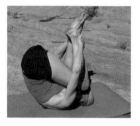

2. Rolling Like a Ball, page 138

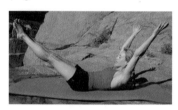

3. Double-Leg Stretch, page 140

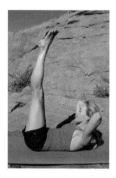

4. Double-Straight-Leg Stretch, page 185

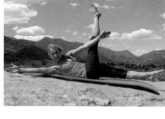

5. Crossover, page 184

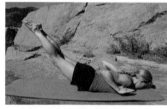

6. Open-Leg Rocker, page 142

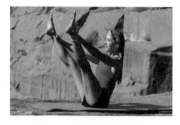

7. Swan Dive or Swan Rocking, page 146 or 191

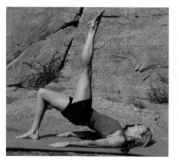

8. Shoulder Bridge with Kicks, page 152

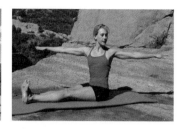

9. Spine Twist, page 153

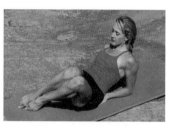

10. Cancan, page 180

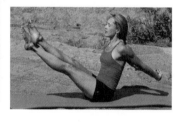

11. Boomerang, page 164

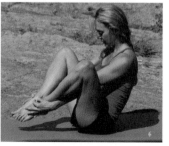

12. Seal, page 166

Pilates Boosts

To boost your training, combine the upper-body exercises from Routines A and B into a single session and add one of the full-body conditioning Pilates routines in Part III to your weekly practice. In the off-season, you may want to consider rock climbing or swimming to maintain upper-body and core fitness. Athletes living in places such as Colorado, Utah, Nevada, New Mexico, and California have access to climbing year-round. Many states without access to year-round outdoor climbing have indoor climbing facilities.

The following section contains Pilates exercises for specific types of paddling. In this section, you will also find after-padding stretches and six tips for incorporating Pilates principles into your paddling.

Boosts for White-Water Paddlers

Whether you are canoeing or kayaking, white water puts additional stress on the body and demands greater fitness and awareness. To boost cross-training fitness, add the following exercises to either Routine A or B.

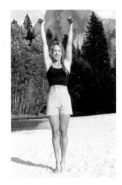

1. Arm Circles, page 194

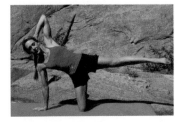

2. Kneeling Side Kicks, page 162

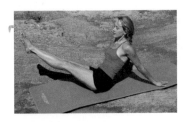

3. Hip Circles, page 158

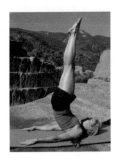

4. Jackknife, page 154

Boosts for Smooth-Water Paddlers

Smooth-water paddlers will benefit from the following additional exercises designed to boost shoulder integrity.

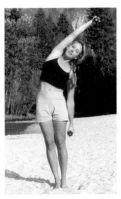

1. Side-to-Side, page 205

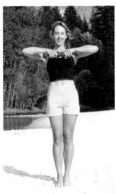

2. Zip-Ups, page 210

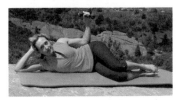

3. Rotator Cuff, page 201

After-Paddling Stretches

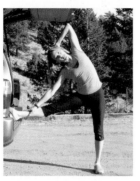

1.
Two-Minute
Tailgate Stretches,
page 218

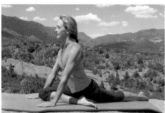

2.
Pigeon Pose,
page 216

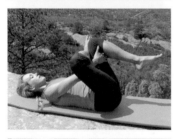

3.
Figure 4,
page 212

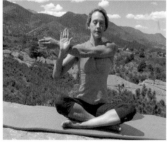

4.
Shoulder
Stretch,
page 218

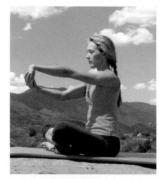

5.
Forearm Stretch,
page 213

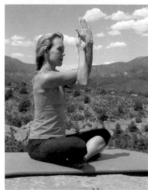

6.
Rhomboid
Stretch,
page 217

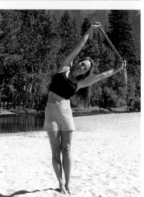

7.
Upper-Body Band
Stretches,
page 219

Pilates in Action:
Six Tips for Paddlers

To maximize the crossover of your skills from the mat to the water, here are six exercises designed to integrate your skills. Choose one at a time and practice them in calm conditions. Once you've gained comfort with all six, keep them in your toolbox as tactics for improving performance.

1. **Breathing:** Breathe deeply. Create a rhythm of breathing and coordinate it with your paddling. For example, depending on the speed of your stroke, you could inhale to pause before a stroke, then exhale deeply as you commit to a stroke.

2. **Centering:** Engage your core. When making powerful strokes, pull your navel to your spine. Stay centered in your core and coordinate the movement of your limbs around your center of gravity.

3. **Concentration:** Strengthen your mind-body connection. Use your breath and intention to keep you centered and present. Practice paddling in a style that is focused on solving the task at hand.

4. **Control:** Calculate the amount of power and strength required for each stroke. Create a dynamic line of energy that transfers power from your lower body through your core to your stroke.

5. **Fluid Motion:** Transition seamlessly from one move to the next. Allow your movement to be fluid and rhythmic. Imagine the shape of each stroke and create a sense of continuous effort so there is no beginning or end.

6. **Precision:** When possible, be more concerned about creating the best possible stroke than about speed. Be quiet and still in your torso and soft in the shoulders, elbows, and jaw. Keep your body centered over your boat and avoid unnecessary movement or tension.

Chapter 10

Road and Trail Runners

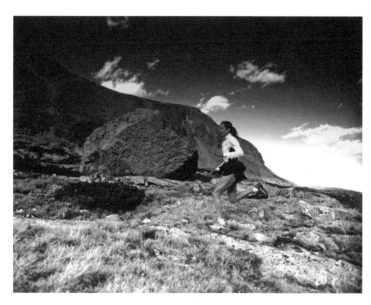

Picture the stride of a strong distance runner. Is it fluid and energy efficient or choppy and wasteful? Chances are it is characterized by vertical alignment from the ears to the ankles, feet landing directly below the body, relaxed shoulders, and steady breathing. A strong runner stabilizes from the core, moves forward landing on the midfoot, and minimizes up-and-down and side-to-side motion. Now envision the stride of a struggling runner. Does she break at the hips, lean too far forward, or bounce up and down? Does she run with tense shoulders, clenched fists, a swayed back, or practice shallow breathing? Chances are good that more energy is being expended, thereby causing more impact. The quality of a runner's posture, fitness, and breathing can mean the difference between a fluid and efficient stride and one that leaves him hobbling.

Cross-Training for a Better Stride

Proper alignment, muscle balance, core strength, and awareness are your tools to a stride that is fast and light. Standing tall with your chest lifted and your body aligned improves movement and breathing. A strong core provides stability for the pelvis and support for the low back. Flexibility in the legs, hips, torso, and shoulders improves range of motion and promotes forward lean from the ankles and not the waist. Balanced muscles in the legs and hips maintain the integrity of your joints and reduce risk of injury. By practicing Pilates regularly, you will be rewarded with a fluid, energy-efficient stride and a more balanced body for years to come. Before diving into the Pilates for Runners routines, it will benefit you in your quest for fitness to become familiar with common overuse injuries and the muscle-balancing requirements of runners.

Overuse Injuries

Below is a list of the most common overuse running injuries that could be prevented through proper warm-ups, cross-training, and rest. For more information about these injuries, please refer to Appendix C.

Feet:
• Achilles Tendonitis
• Fallen Metatarsal Arch
• Plantar Fasciitis

Ankles:
• Ankle Sprains

Lower Leg:
• Shin Splints

Knees:
• Chondromalacia
• Meniscus Injuries
• Patella Tendonitis
  (Jumper's Knee)
• Patellofemoral Pain Syndrome
  (Runner's Knee)
• Plica Syndrome

Upper Leg:
• Iliotibial Band Syndrome

Hips:
• Arthritis
• Bursitis
• Tendonitis
• Stress Fractures

Back:
• Sciatica

If you have a history of running injuries, it is worthwhile to consider your alignment, shoes, running stride, and training practices.

Alignment

The alignment of your feet affects the integrity of your ankle, knee, and hip joints. Like a tall building, if the bottom floor collapses, every floor above is compromised. In addition to faulty foot mechanics, leg length discrepancies, legs that bow, knock knees, high Q-angles, and scoliosis can all create misalignments. Clues that one leg is longer than the other include the sole of one shoe wearing out more quickly than the other or one shoulder that is higher than the other. The shoe with the most wear indicates the longer leg, while the higher shoulder is often the side with the shorter leg. The shoulder lifts in an attempt to keep your body aligned. If you suspect alignment issues, seek a professional analysis and purchase appropriate footwear or arch support.

Shoes

Purchase your shoes from a store where the staff is knowledgeable and can recommend appropriate footwear for your foot type and running habits. For example, some shoes are designed to give extra support to a foot that overpronates. If your foot underpronates and you wear such shoes, they can cause an injury to your foot and legs. When buying shoes, consider three factors: your foot, your stride, and your leg characteristics. First, do you overpronate or underpronate? Second, is your stride long, short, or somewhere in between? Third, do your legs bow, knock-knee, or have a high Q-angle? Women runners with wide hips have higher Q-angles. (The quadriceps angle is measured by a line drawn from the front side of your hip bone [the anterior superior iliac spine] to the center of your kneecap, and another line drawn from the center of your kneecap to just below where the patellar tendon inserts.)

Replacing footwear on a timely basis is equally important. After the first 300 to 500 miles of running, most shoes lose 60 percent of their shock absorption. If you are running 15 miles per week, plan on replacing your shoes every 6 to 8 months. Trail runners may even consider running shoes specifically designed for trails. These shoes offer less cushioning but deliver more traction and support.

Stride

The average runner takes approximately 2,000 strides in a mile. If you run five miles three times a week, that's 30,000 times that you land on your feet. With each stride, your feet, knees, and hips absorb three to four times your body weight. If you weigh 150 pounds, that equates to landing with 600 pounds of force on your muscles, joints, and bones. The impact of running creates more overuse injuries than any other outdoor sport.

Additionally, the faster you run, the greater the impact. Runners who swing their feet forward and backward, creating a large pendulum of recovery and strike through the heel, increase impact and reduce efficiency. In addition, up-and-down and side-to-side motion should be minimized, as the emphasis should be on forward motion. Track your feet, knees, ankles, and shoulders forward as if they were moving over two invisible rails.

Training Practices

For many, running is an activity that transcends exercise and becomes a meditation. However, running too much, too intensely, or failing to cross-train can lead to injury. As is true with other sports, it is best not to increase your mileage, speed, or intensity by more than 10 percent in a week. In fact, you should only increase one of the three factors in a given week. Remember: overuse injuries result from the decisions we make over time. By using appropriate footwear and practicing smart training, you will improve your stride, muscle balance, and the integrity of your joints.

7 Tips for Avoiding Injury

1. Before running, warm up by walking at a fast pace. After your run, do post-running stretches.

2. Maintain muscle balance in your legs and hips.

3. Avoid running beyond your current skills and fitness.

4. While running, keep your weight centered over your hips and maintain good alignment of your legs.

5. Maintain good posture while running. Keep your hips level, lengthen your torso, and keep your chest open.

6. Follow the 10 percent rule. Avoid increasing interval training, mileage, or frequency by more than 10 percent in a given week.

7. Listen to your body and learn to identify the difference between good muscle soreness and pain. If you feel pain, identify its location, what activity seemed to cause it, and monitor any changes. If the pain persists, see a qualified professional before it becomes chronic.

Creating Balance

Running recruits heavily from the hamstrings, hip flexors, and calves. This results in tightness and weakness in the medial quadriceps, adductors, and hip extensors. These muscle imbalances place unequal tension on the cartilage, tendons, and ligaments that support the hips, knees, and feet. Over time the joints become compromised and unstable. Muscle imbalances and joint instability can also occur from trail running over sloping terrain, running too often, or favoring one leg as you stride. Muscle imbalances occur not only from the front to back, but also from left to right. This creates stress all the way into the lower back. An effective Pilates cross-training routine focuses on boosting core strength, restoring muscle balance, and improving flexibility. Please note that some muscles may fall into both categories.

MUSCLES TO STRETCH AND STRENGTHEN

	STRETCH	STRENGTHEN
Lower Body	Quadriceps	Medial Quadriceps
	Hamstrings	Shins (Tibialis Anterior)
	Calves (Gastronemius and Soleus)	
	Iliotibial Band	
Core	Quadratus Lumborum	Abdominals
	Hip Flexors	Hip Extensors
	Hip Abductors	Hip Adductors
Upper Body	Pectorals	Pectorals
	Upper Trapezius	Rhomboids
	Neck Extensors	Mid- and Lower Trapezius
	Latissimus Dorsi	Latissimus Dorsi
	Serratus Anterior	

15-Minute Pilates Prescription

The beauty of Pilates exercises is that you can simultaneously stretch one part of your body while strengthening another part. On the following pages are two 15-minute routines. They are designed to meet the cross-training needs of a runner. Alternate between the two routines during your practice three to five times a week. For a complete 30- to 45-minute full-body general-conditioning Pilates workout, refer to the classical routines presented in Part III. For all routines, exercise descriptions are provided in Part III: Your Toolbox. The exercises are ordered in a way that adheres most closely to the Classical Mat Sequence. The sequence is designed to warm up the body and spine and create a satisfying and continuous flow of movement. Use these pages as a reference. I encourage you to make a copy for easy use when cross-training at the gym or on a trip.

One Size Doesn't Fit All

Running surface, distance, and frequency influence your training needs. Running over sloping, rocky, and slippery surfaces requires more agility and upper-body fitness than running on a flat surface. No matter what type of running you prefer, core strength, flexibility, and uniform muscle development are key. This triad creates a foundation for performing your best and avoiding injury. By no means should you feel compelled to do only the following routines. This book contains more than 80 exercises, enabling you to create a variety of routines to meet your needs. If you choose to design your own routine, use your SWOT self-analysis from Chapter 4 for guidance and refer to the Pilates Exercise Reference Chart in Appendix A. Use the worksheet in Appendix B to create your own Pilates prescription.

Pilates for Runners

Goal:

Boost core strength

Uniformly balance muscles

Improve flexibility

Formula:

Strengthen the abdominal and back muscles

Strengthen non-running muscles (antagonists)

Stretch running muscles (agonists)

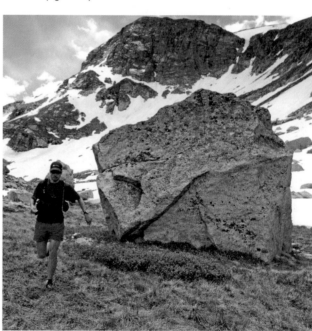

Routine A

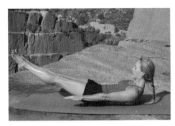

1. The Hundred, page 130

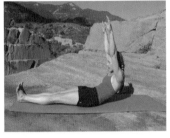

2. Roll Up, page 132

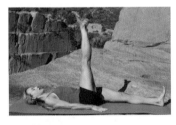

3. One-Leg Circles, page 136

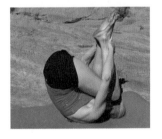

4. Rolling Like a Ball, page 138

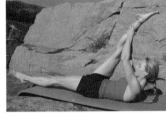

5. One-Straight-Leg Stretch, page 188

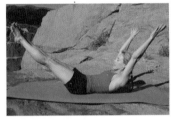

6. Double-Leg Stretch, page 140

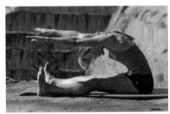

7. Spine Stretch, page 141

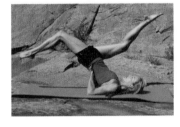

8. Bicycle, page 151

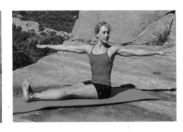

9. Spine Twist, page 153

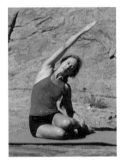

10. T-Bird, page 192

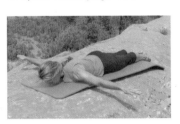

11. Mermaid, page 215

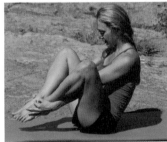

12. Seal, page 166

Routine B

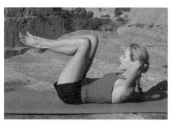

1. Footwork, page 187

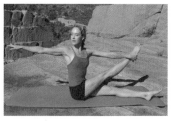

2. Tree, page 193

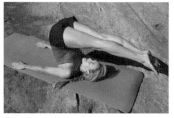

3. Roll Over, page 134

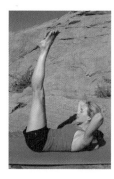

4. Double-Straight-Leg
Stretch, page 185

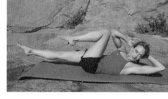

5. Crisscross, page 183

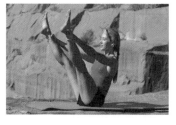

6. Open-Leg Rocker, page 142

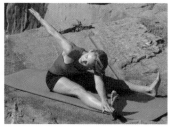

7. Saw, page 145

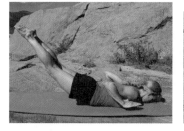

8. Swan Dive or Swan
Rocking, page 146 or 191

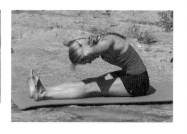

9. Neck Pull, page 149

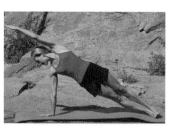

10. Side Bend, page 163

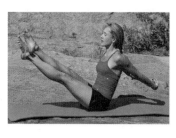

11. Boomerang, page 164

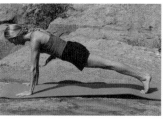

12. Push-Ups, page 168

Pilates Boosts

To boost your training, add one of the full-body conditioning Pilates routines from Part III to your weekly practice. In the off-season, you may want to consider cross-country skiing or snowshoeing. Soft snow makes for a low-impact workout that's easy on the knees. It will not only keep your legs strong, it will keep your cardio-vascular fitness tuned and improve upper-body strength for trail running.

The following section contains Pilates exercises for specific types of running. In this section, you will also find after-running stretches and six tips for incorporating Pilates principles into your running.

Boosts for Trail Running

Running trails puts stress your lower body in ways road running doesn't. Alignment, muscle balance, and core strength become even more imperative to avoid injury. In addition, upper-body fitness helps you power up hills and provides counterbalance for the lower body. Trail running requires you to be agile, adaptable, and masterful at minimizing impact. The benefits of trail running include increased endurance and confidence. As you continuously adapt to the ups and downs, slopes, and obstacles along a trail, your cardiovascular fitness is strengthened. Core strength adds support to the lower back but also minimizes impact on the spine and knees. If you enjoy running trails, add the following exercises to either Routine A or B.

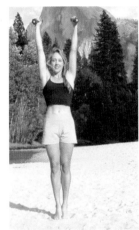

1.
Arm
Circles,
page 194

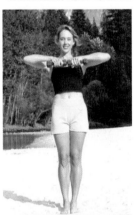

2.
Zip-Ups,
page 210

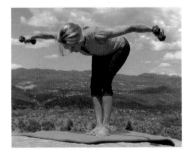

3. Bug, page 195

After-Running Stretches

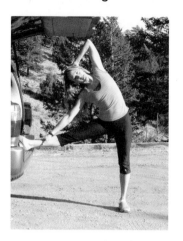

1. Two-Minute Tailgate Stretches, page 218

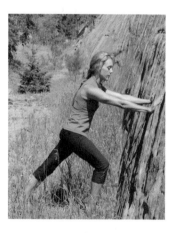

2. Calves Stretch, page 211

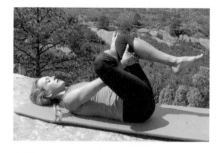

3. Figure 4, page 212

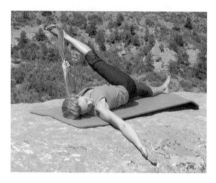

4. Leg Stretch with Band, page 214

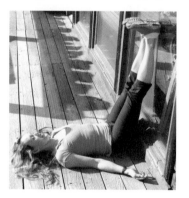

5. Wall Stretch, page 220

Pilates in Action:
Six Tips for Runners

To maximize the crossover of your skills from the mat to the trail, here are six exercises designed to leverage your movement skills while running. Choose one at a time and practice them on a run. Once you've gained comfort with all six, put them on your checklist while running.

1. **Breathing:** Breathe deeply. Create a rhythm of breathing and coordinate it with your stride. By inhaling through the nose and exhaling through the mouth, you'll stay dialed-in to your heart rate and exertion levels and dehydrate less quickly. Because nose breathing stimulates the parasympathetic nervous system, you'll feel calmer.

2. **Centering:** Engage your core by pulling your navel to your spine. Pretend your running shorts have a zipper that is holding in your abdomen firmly. This will help you to engage your core, provide support for your lower back, and minimize excessive torso rotation.

3. **Concentration:** Strengthen your mind-body connection. Practice a running style that is focused on staying relaxed in the shoulders and core-centered to reduce impact and increase efficiency of stride.

4. **Control:** Calculate the amount of energy and strength required for each stride. Maintain good posture and form.

5. **Flowing Motion:** Fluid, energy-efficient strides make running feel effortless. Allow your stride to carry you forward like a flowing river, and minimize the up-and-down motion. Push through the big toe to propel you and feel as though you are gently leaning forward.

6. **Precision:** Challenge yourself to run as softly as possible and minimize the impact on your body. The quieter you can run, the softer and more energy-efficient your stride will be. Pretend as though you have a string connected from your second toe to your knee to your hip and keep them all connected in the same line as you stride.

Chapter 11

Skiers and Snowboarders

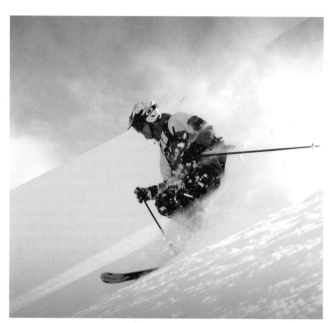

What once served as a mode of transportation in Scandinavian countries centuries ago has since evolved into a diverse and world-famous sport. Today, there are two main disciplines of skiing: Nordic (cross-country and Telemark) and alpine. Although they differ in technical style and equipment binding systems, they share a downhill forward stance and require similar fitness. Cross-country skiing is differentiated into classical and skate skiing. Classical skiing movement is similar to a running stride, whereas skate skiing is similar to speed skating or Rollerblading. The legs push outward rather than backward and require more lateral hip strength. Both are similar in that they use poles to propel forward motion.

Over the past 40 years, snowboarding began carving out a path on the slopes, adding options for alpine skiers. Like skiers, boarders choose equipment designed for their style of riding. Three main categories exist: freestyle, free ride, and alpine. Snowboarding differs from skiing in that it utilizes a side stance and a binding system without releases. Skiers maintain even weight over their feet and alternate pressure from right and left, inside and out as they turn, whereas boarders maintain more weight on either the front or back foot, depending on the snow conditions. This creates more-significant muscle imbalances from left to right. Whether you are skiing or boarding, both require proper alignment, lower-body fitness, core strength, and a strong mind-body connection.

Stacking Your Bones

Keeping the torso upright while stacking the ankles, knees, hips, and shoulders over the center of your board(s) with slightly flexed knees produces better alignment and technique. Alignment helps skiers and boarders apply pressure through the feet to turn and maintain a quiet torso, thereby improving balance, agility, and breathing.

Tightening Your Core

If you spend any time on double-black diamond runs where moguls become monsters, you'll appreciate the additional core strength gained from Pilates. Skiers and boarders recruit power from the hips and core. Skiers rely on a lateral side-to-side hip movement to access the inside and outside edge of the ski. Boarders rely on tipping their hips forward and back to access the toe-side and heel-side edge. In addition, boarders use more rotational movement to change directions. Tapping into a strong core, you'll improve your balance, agility, and be more in control. Integrating core strength into your edging, you'll transfer a powerful line

of energy to your skis or board. By tightening your core, you'll reduce impact on your back, hips, and knees. Since core strength improves balance, you may also find yourself falling less. Being agile and adaptable at high speeds, in changing snow conditions, with varying steepness of runs, and among obstacles such as trees, moguls, and people is common to skiers and boarders alike.

As you improve your alignment and core strength, your movements become energy efficient, minimize wear and tear on your joints, and are more enjoyable. Before diving into the Pilates for Skiers and Boarders routines, it will benefit you in your quest for fitness and longevity to address common overuse injuries and the training needs of skiers and boarders.

Overuse Injuries

Over the past 20 years, ski injuries have declined with the advent of shorter, shaped skis. However, snowboarding injuries have risen. This is primarily due to the growth in the sport. Unless you like to live on the edge or are a machismo first-timer opting out of a lesson, your chances of getting injured snowboarding are no greater than they are skiing.

Following is a list of the most common overuse injuries to skiers and boarders. Falling is the primary reason for many injuries, especially to the shoulders and knees. While some injuries are more common to skiers (knee injuries) and others to boarders (ankle injuries), shoulder injuries sustained by falling occur equally between the two types of athletes. For more information about these injuries, please refer to Appendix C.

Feet:
• Achilles Tendonitis
• Talus Injuries
Ankles:
• Ankle Sprains
Knees:
• Anterior Cruciate Ligament (ACL) Injury
• Chondromalacia
• Medial Collateral Ligament (MCL) Injury
• Meniscus Injuries

• Patellofemoral Pain Syndrome (Runner's Knee)
• Patella Tendonitis (Jumper's Knee)
Legs:
• Shin Splints
• Iliotibial Band Syndrome
Back:
• Sciatica
Shoulders:
• AC (Acromioclavicular) Joint Separations
• Broken Collarbones
• Shoulder Dislocations
Hands:
• Ulnar Collateral Ligament Injury (Skier's Thumb)
• Wrist Fractures
Neck:
• Whiplash

Most injuries manifest over time as the result of bad technique, improperly fitting gear, or poor fitness. Movement that is sloppy, careless, tense, inefficient, or out of control places wear and tear on your joints and increases your odds of falling. Improperly fitted equipment, bad form, structural misalignments, muscle imbalances, and going from couch to cliff are just a few of the ways skiers and boarders get injured.

Super-Sized Equipment

Skis or boards that are too long and improperly fitted boots can lead to injury. When buying equipment, consider three factors: your foot, your ability, and your intentions. First, does your foot over- or under-pronate? Depending on the structure of your foot, you many want to consider arch supports. Second, are you a beginner, intermediate, or expert? Third, what type of skiing or riding do you plan to do and in what conditions?

From Couch to Cliff

Going from couch to cliff without any preparation or taking too many runs in the preseason is a formula for injury. Likewise, keep in mind that while you may be prepared, others may not be. The exhilaration of fresh powder and crisp air draws millions of skiers and snowboarders to the mountains each year. Therefore, maintaining good fitness and a strong mind-body connection will help keep you safer. As mentioned in previous chapters, it is best to build up your volume and intensity gradually. Give yourself time to build your fitness and confidence before taking on the double-diamonds. Pilates will help you start the ski season with balanced muscles and maintain them through-out the season.

Keep Your Balance

Overly developed quadriceps muscles, underdeveloped hamstrings, and inner and outer thighs can stress the soft tissues around the knees and make them unstable. Snowboarders experience muscle imbalance not only from the front to the back but also from the right to left leg due to the side stance. Muscle imbalances can also be caused by structural misalign-ments such as leg-length discrepancy, legs that bow, knock-knees, or a high Q-angle. (The quadriceps angle is measured by a line drawn from the front side of your hip bone [the anterior superior iliac spine] to the center of your kneecap, and another line drawn from the center of your kneecap to just below where the patellar tendon inserts.) You'll reduce your chances for injury by improving the alignment of your feet, knees, and hips. You can often correct structural misalignments with proper footwear and arch supports.

Falling

Many injuries manifest through falling. Although falling is often a necessary part of learning, high-speed falls or those delivering great impact increase your odds of injury. When taking a fall, don't get up until you've stopped sliding. If you try to resist the direction your skis or board are traveling, you may create a twisting motion on your knees. Falling can cause shoulder injuries such as dislocations, collarbone fractures, and AC (acromioclavicular) joint separation. Unless your equipment fails or someone runs you down, muscle fatigue, insufficient skill, loss of balance, skiing too fast, and mental fatigue all contribute to falls. Improving your strength, flexibility, alignment, core strength, and mind-body connection won't eliminate falls, but they will make your body more resilient. By practicing Pilates, you'll be more in tune with your body, know your limits, and thereby have a better chance of staying injury free.

7 Tips for Avoiding Injury

1. Warm up on easy slopes and stretch the quadriceps and hamstrings to reduce pressure on the knee.

2. Maintain muscle balance in your legs and hips.

3. While skiing or boarding, keep your weight centered over your hips.

4. Maintain good posture.

5. Follow the 10 percent rule. Choose to increase only one of the following factors by 10 percent in a given week: intensity, frequency, or volume.

6. Avoid runs beyond your current skills and fitness.

7. Listen to your body. Go home when you're tired. If you feel pain, identify its location, what activity seemed to cause it, and monitor any changes. If the pain persists, see a qualified professional before it becomes chronic.

Skiers and Snowboarders

107

THE PILATES PRESCRIPTION: 15 MINUTES A DAY

Creating Balance

An effective Pilates cross-training routine focuses on boosting core strength, improving flexibility, and restoring muscle balance. To create a Pilates cross-training program that restores muscle balance and joint integrity, let's identify the skiing/ boarding muscles that require stretching and the skiing/boarding muscles that need strengthening. Please note that some muscles may require both strengthening and stretching.

MUSCLES TO STRETCH AND STRENGTHEN

	STRETCH	STRENGTHEN
Lower Body	Quadriceps	Medial Quadriceps
	Hamstrings	Hamstrings
	Illiotibial Band	
	Calves (Gastronemius and Soleus)	Shins (Tibialis Anterior)
Core	Quadratus Lumborum	Abdominals
	Hip Abductors	Hip Adductors
	Hip Flexors	Hip Abductors
	Hip Extensors	Hip Extensors
Upper Body	Pectorals	Rhomboids
	Upper Trapezius	Mid-Trapezius
	Latissmus Dorsi	Lower Trapezius

15-Minute Pilates Prescription

The beauty of Pilates exercises is that you can simultaneously stretch one part of your body while strengthening another part. On the following pages are two 15-minute routines. They are designed to meet the cross-training needs of a skier or snowboarder. Alternate between the two routines during your practice three to five times a week. For a complete 30- to 45-minute full-body general-conditioning Pilates workout, refer to the classical routines presented in Part III. For all routines, exercise descriptions are provided in Part III: Your Toolbox. The exercises are ordered in a way that adheres most closely to the Classical Mat Sequence. The sequence is designed to warm up the body and spine and create a satisfying and continuous flow of movement. Use these pages as a reference. I encourage you to make a copy for easy use when cross-training at the gym or on a trip.

One Size Doesn't Fit All

Whether you like to ski or board the moguls, powder, or groomers, factors that influence your training needs include the terrain, your frequency, and level of challenge. No matter your preference, core strength, flexibility, and uniform muscle development are key. This triad creates a foundation for performing your best and avoiding injury. By no means should you feel compelled to do only the following routines. This book contains more than 80 exercises, enabling you to create a variety of routines to suit your needs. If you choose to design your own routine, use your SWOT self-analysis from Chapter 4 for guidance and refer to the Pilates Exercise Reference Chart in Appendix A. Use the worksheet in Appendix B to create your own Pilates prescription.

Pilates for Skiers and Snowboarders

Goal:

Boost core strength

Uniformly balance muscles

Improve flexibility

Formula:

Strengthen the abdominal and back muscles

Strengthen non-skiing/boarding muscles (antagonists)

Stretch skiing/boarding muscles (agonists)

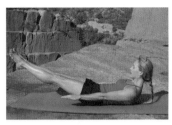

1. The Hundred, page 130

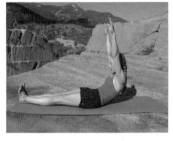

2. Roll Up, page 132

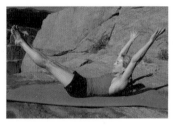

3. One-Leg Stretch, page 139

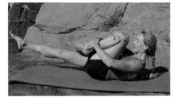

4. Double-Leg Stretch, page 140

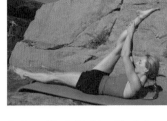

5. One-Straight-Leg Stretch, page 188

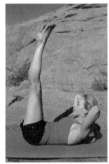

6. Double-Straight-Leg Stretch, page 185

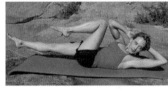

7. Crisscross, page 183

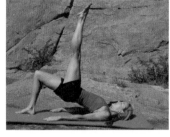

8. Shoulder Bridge with Kicks, page 152

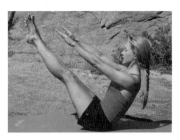

9. Teaser Series, page 156

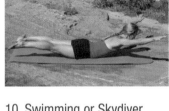

10. Swimming or Skydiver, page 159 or 189

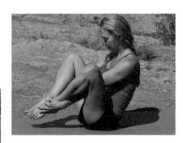

11. Seal, page 166

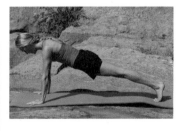

12. Push-Ups, page 168

Routine B

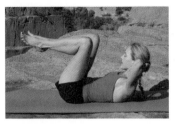

1. Footwork, page 187

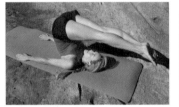

2. Roll Over, page 134

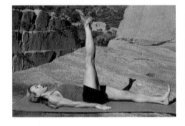

3. One-Leg Circles, page 136

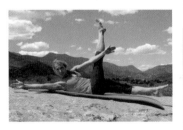

4. Crossover, page 184

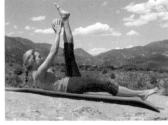

5. Captain Crunch, page 181

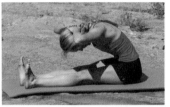

6. Neck Pull, page 149

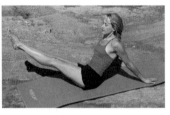

7. Hip Circles or Cancan, page 158 or 180

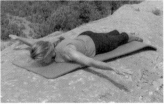

8. T-Bird, page 192

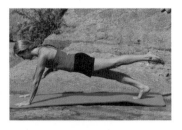

9. Leg Pull-Front, page 160

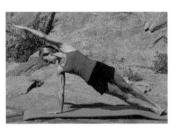

10. Side Bend, page 163

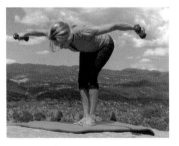

11. Bug, page 195

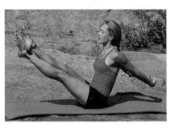

12. Boomerang, page 164

Pilates Boosts

To boost your training, combine the leg and hip exercises from Routines A and B into a single session and add one of the full-body conditioning Pilates routines in Part III to your weekly practice. In the off-season, you may want to consider trail running. It will not only keep your legs strong, it will keep your cardio-vascular fitness tuned and improve upper-body strength.

The following section contains Pilates exercises for specific types of skiing or boarding. Once you have gained confidence with Routines A and B, add these exercises, if appropriate. In this section, you will also find end-of-the-day stretches and six tips for incorporating Pilates principles while skiing or boarding.

Boosts for Cross-Country Skiers

Classical skiing movement is similar to a running stride, whereas skate skiing is similar to speed skating or Rollerblading. In skate skiing, the legs push outward rather than backward and require more lateral hip strength. Both are similar in that they use poles to propel forward motion. To boost leg, core, and upper-body strength, add the following exercises to your cross-training routine:

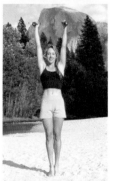

1. Corkscrew, page 144

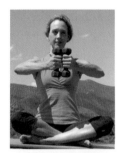

2. Triceps Kickbacks, page 208

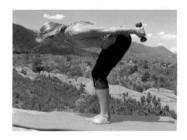

3. Hug a Tree, page 200

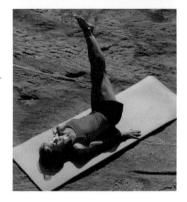

4. Arm Circles, page 194

Boosts for Snowboarders

To balance out right- and left-leg muscle imbalances created from the side stance of snowboarding, consider doubling the number of leg exercise repetitions on your less-dominant snowboarding leg. The less-dominant side is the one that typically sustains less weight. Also add the following exercises to your routine:

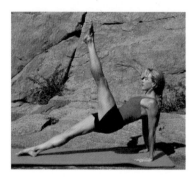

1. Kneeling Side Kicks, page 162

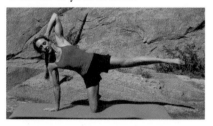

2. Leg Pull-Up, page 161

After-Skiing/-Snowboarding Stretches

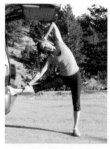

1. Two-Minute Tailgate Stretches, page 218

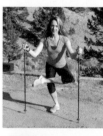

2. Figure 4 with Ski Poles or Hiking Poles, page 213

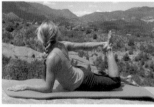

3. Quadriceps Stretch, page 217

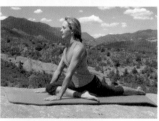

4. Pigeon Pose, page 216

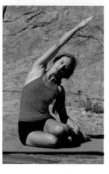

5. Mermaid, page 215

Pilates in Action: Six Tips for Skiers and Snowboarders

To maximize the crossover of your skills from the mat to the slopes, try the following exercises on an easy run that is well below your ability:

1. **Breathing:** Create more awareness of the use of breath. Breathe deeply. Create a rhythm of breathing and coordinate it with your turns.

2. **Centering:** Engage your core. Pull your navel to your spine and narrow your waist like an hourglass. You'll improve your center of gravity in your hips, support your lower back, and minimize torso rotation.

3. **Concentration:** Strengthen your mind-body connection. Practice skiing/boarding in a style that is focused on solving the task at hand. Choose one technique and work on refining it during the course of a run.

4. **Control:** Ski or board in control. Know where your edge is and work within this framework.

5. **Fluid Motion:** Create movement that is fluid and rhythmic. Transition seamlessly from one turn to the next. Allow your turns to carry you forward like a steady river and minimize the up-and-down motion.

6. **Precision:** Challenge yourself to be precise in your alignment, weight distribution, and edging techniques.

Chapter 12

Multisport: Write Your Own Ticket

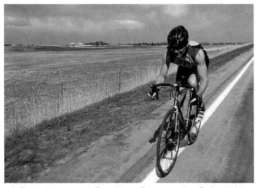

Richard Rossiter near Boulder Reservoir, Colorado.

According to USA Triathlon, an organization that promotes multisports in the United States, between 150,000 and 250,000 people in the United States participate in multisport events each year. Multisport events encompass everything from traditional triathlons, duathlons, and biathlons to events that include alpine and Nordic skiing, mountain biking, paddle sports, orienteering, and even climbing. Some races challenge the individual while others are team sports and relays. Duathlons (run-cycle-run events), aquathlons (swim and run), winter triathlon (running, mountain biking, and cross-country skiing, all on snow), and sprint-distance triathlons are popular events sweeping the nation. Multisport events are as diverse as the athlete and draw people from all walks of life. What they have in common is that they all require physical and mental endurance.

Training for a multisport event can be as time consuming as holding a part-time job. Whether your goal is to do an Ironman in Hawaii, an Eco-Challenge, or a local sprint-distance triathlon, Pilates cross-training is an integral part of performing your best and staying injury free. By squeezing in as little as 15 minutes of Pilates three to five days a week, you'll experience better movement, suppler muscles, and reduce your risk of injury.

Aligning for Efficiency

Alignment is the cornerstone of athletic performance. The tools for improving alignment are awareness, core strength, flexibility, and muscle balance. Alignment improves the quality and energy efficiency of all your movements. When the bones are properly aligned, work is reduced on the muscles and more efficiency is created in the body. Proper alignment takes stress off your joints, increases ease of movement, and improves breathing. For a swimmer, proper alignment is fundamental to an energy-efficient stroke. Maintaining a streamlined position, rotating your hips and shoulders around your spine, and breathing bilaterally (from both the left side and right side) are enhanced through alignment. As a result you roll more easily, experience less drag, and improve power and speed. For a cyclist, better alignment creates a more aerodynamic position, improves pedal cadence, and reduces stress on the shoulders, neck, and lower back. For a runner, better alignment reduces energy expenditure, creates less stress on the knees, hips, and back, and improves your stride.

Building Blocks

A strong core improves alignment, balance, and power. For a swimmer, a strong core improves long-axis rotation by transferring power from the upper body to the lower body. For a cyclist, core strength stabilizes the torso and improves pedal power when standing and pulling on the handlebars. For a runner, a strong core supports good posture, stride, and reduces the risk of lower-back injury.

Flexibility is also essential to the multisport athlete. Flexibility improves joint range of motion and ease of movement. Flexibility improves torso rotation while swimming, aerodynamics and comfort while cycling, and muscle resiliency while running.

No matter what the sport, uniform muscle balance bolsters joint integrity. Balanced muscles—front to back, medially and laterally, and left to right—are strong, flexible, and resilient. Strengthening under-used muscles and stretching overused muscles reduce risk of injury to your shoulders while swimming and to your knees, hips, and back while cycling and running.

Breath:
The Mind-Body Bridge

Proper alignment opens the way to better breathing. Breathing is the bridge between the mind and body and the fuel for muscular endurance, allowing you to perform your best. Deep breathing allows you to maximize lung capacity, minimize energy expenditure, and improve cardiovascular endurance. Steady breathing reduces the accumulation of lactic acid in your muscles and keeps you focused and calm. If you are participating in a triathlon race that can require treading water for 10 or 15 minutes, you'll appreciate the calming effect of conscious breathing.

In your quest for fitness, it will benefit you to address the most common overuse injuries and the muscle-balance needs of a multisport athlete.

Overuse Injuries

If you have aspirations to compete in an event that requires many qualifying activities, you cannot afford to be injured. The most common injuries to multisport athletes affect the knees, lower legs, ankles, feet, lower back, and shoulders. Many injuries can be prevented by incorporating Pilates cross-training into your weekly routine. Below are the most common injuries in multisport athletes. For more information about these injuries, please refer to Appendix C.

Feet:
• Achilles Tendonitis
• Plantar Fasciitis

Lower Leg:
• Shin Splints

Knees:
• Chondromalacia
• Patellofemoral Pain Syndrome (Runner's Knee)
• Patella Tendonitis (Jumper's Knee)

Upper Leg:
• Iliotibial Band Syndrome

Back:
• Sciatica

Shoulders:
• Rotator Cuff Tendonitis (Swimmer's Shoulder)

Multisport athletes experience overuse injuries for a variety of reasons, including poor alignment, fitness, and training practices.

THE PILATES PRESCRIPTION: 15 MINUTES A DAY

Out of Line

Poor alignment makes achieving good form and energy efficiency next to impossible. It can be caused by improp–erly fitted gear such as a bike that doesn't fit, running shoes that are too small, or lack of adequate arch support.

Pilates can't help much with equipment problems; however, other common causes of poor alignment can also be structural misalignments, including faulty foot biomechanics, curvature of the spine, and one leg that is longer than the other. Bad posture, poor sports movements, and inadequate fitness are equally culpable and are areas that may be addressed by incorporating a consistent Pilates routine.

Irrespective of the cause, misalignment has a rippling effect on the body. For a swimmer, poor alignment makes it difficult to roll the torso and puts excess stress on the shoulders. For a cyclist and runner, poor alignment increases the risk of injury to the knees and hips.

Overuse

The more you train, the greater your risk of injury. Consider that the average competitive swimmer rotates his shoulder as many as a million times in a given week and that a runner may stride more than 30,000 times in an average week. Overusing muscles can result in insufficient lubrication of the joints and lead to injuries such as

bursitis. Such repetitive motion makes proper muscle balance a priority. For a swimmer, muscle imbalances in the shoulders and upper back can result in swimmer's shoulder. For cyclists and runners, imbalances in the legs and hips lead to a variety of knee injuries. As stated in previous chapters, training mistakes such as increasing volume, intensity, or duration by more than 10 percent in a week are an easy way to create injury.

7 Tips for Avoiding Injury

1. Warm up and stretch.

2. Maintain muscle balance in your lower and upper body.

3. Avoid participating in events that are beyond your skills and fitness.

4. Use equipment that is properly fitted to your body.

5. Maintain good posture and alignment while training.

6. Follow the 10 percent rule. Choose to increase only one of the following factors by 10 percent in a given week: intensity, frequency, or volume.

7. Listen to your body and learn to identify the difference between good muscle soreness and pain. If you feel pain, identify its location, what activity seemed to cause it, and monitor any changes. If the pain persists, see a qualified professional before it becomes chronic.

Creating Balance

In the course of this book, we have addressed the cross-training needs of a variety of athletes. The cross-training needs of a multisport athlete encompass many of these sports. Therefore, let's identify for a multisport athlete the most common muscles that require stretching and the muscles that require strengthening. Depending on the specific sports in which you participate, your needs may vary. I encourage you to review the sports-specific chapters that apply to you. Please note that some muscles may require both strengthening and stretching.

MUSCLES TO STRETCH AND STRENGTHEN

	STRETCH	STRENGTHEN
Upper Body	Biceps	Biceps
	Triceps	Triceps
	Pectorals	Pectorals
	Latissimus Dorsi	Latissimus Dorsi
	Upper Trapezius	Mid- and Lower Trapezius
		Rotator Cuff
	Rhomboids	Rhomboids
Core	Hip Flexors	Abdominals
	Hip Extensors	Hip Extensors
	Quadratus Lumborum	Quadratus Lumborum
	Hip Abductors	Hip Adductors
	Hip Adductors	Hip Abductors
Lower Body	Quadriceps	Hamstrings
	Hamstrings	Calves (Gastronemius and Soleus)
	Iliotibial Band	Shins (Tibialis Anterior)

15-Minute Pilates Prescription

The beauty of Pilates exercises is that you can simultaneously stretch one part of your body while strengthening another part. On the following pages are two 15-minute routines. They are designed to meet the cross-training needs of a multisport athlete. Alternate between the two routines during your practice three to five times a week. For a complete 30- to 45-minute full-body general-conditioning Pilates workout, refer to the classical routines presented in Part III. For all routines, exercise descriptions are provided in Part III: Your Toolbox. The exercises are ordered in a way that adheres most closely to the Classical Mat Sequence. The sequence is designed to warm up the body and spine and create a satisfying and continuous flow of movement. Use these pages as a reference. I encourage you to make a copy for easy use when cross-training at the gym or on a trip.

One Size Doesn't Fit All

By no means should you feel compelled to do only the following routines. This book contains more than 80 exercises, enabling you to create a variety of routines to meet your needs. Identifying the muscular demands of your sports is the first step to creating a Pilates cross-training routine.

If you are predisposed to certain injuries or train heavier in one sport than another, consult the Creating Balance section of the chapters that apply to your sports. If you choose to design your own routine, use your SWOT self-analysis for additional guidance and refer to the Pilates Exercise Reference Chart in Appendix A. Use the worksheet in Appendix B to create your own Pilates prescription.

The following Pilates routines are designed for a traditional multisport athlete who is engaging in swimming, cycling, and running.

Pilates for the
Multisport Athlete

Goal:

Boost core strength

Uniformly balance muscles

Improve flexibility

Formula:

Strengthen the abdominal and back muscles

Strengthen supporting muscles (antagonists)

Stretch overworked muscles (agonists)

Routine A

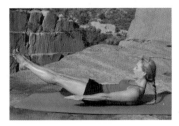

1. The Hundred, page 130

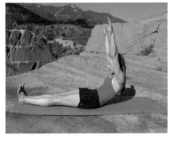

2. Roll Up, page 132

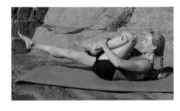

3. One-Leg Stretch, page 139

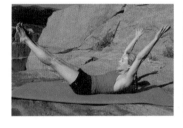

4. Double-Leg Stretch, page 140

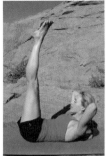

5. Double-Straight-Leg Stretch, page 185

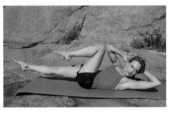

6. Crisscross, page 183

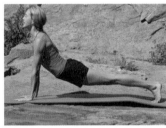

7. Snake, page 190

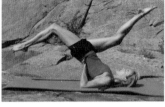

8. Bicycle, page 151

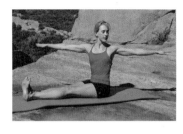

9. Spine Twist, page 153

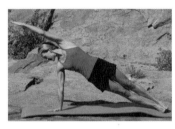

10. Side Bend, page 163

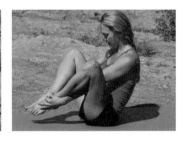

11. Seal, page 166

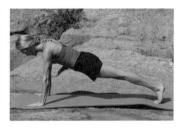

12. Push-Ups, page 168

Routine B

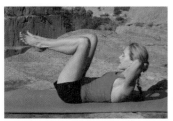

1. Footwork, page 187

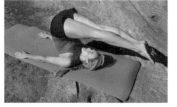

2. Roll Over, page 134

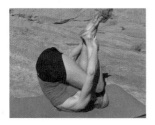

3. Rolling Like a Ball, page 138

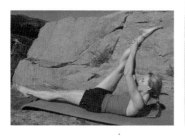

4. One-Straight-Leg Stretch, page 188

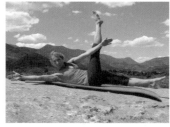

5. Crossover, page 184

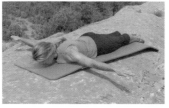

6. T-Bird, page 192

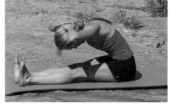

7. Neck Pull, page 149

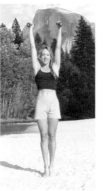

8. Arm Circles, page 194

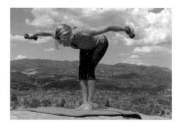

9. Bug, page 195

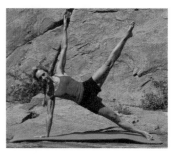

10. Star, page 207

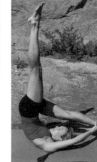

11. Control Balance, page 167

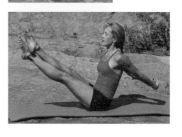

12. Boomerang, page 164

Pilates Boosts

To boost your training, combine exercises from Routines A and B into a single session and add one of the full-body conditioning Pilates routines in Part III to your weekly practice. In the off-season, you may want to consider cross-country skiing or snowshoeing. Soft snow makes for a low-impact workout that's easy on the knees. It will not only keep your legs strong, it will keep your cardio-vascular fitness tuned and, by adding poles, you will improve upper-body strength for trail running.

Boosts for Swimmers

Maintaining strength and flexibility in the shoulders, chest, and mid-back creates better rotation, a longer stroke, and reduces risk of injury. Maintaining a streamlined position tightens the muscles along the spine; Pilates rolling exercises will help. Kicking from the hip utilizes the quadriceps and hips. In addition, the calves work hard to point the toes and minimize drag as you kick. The gluteus muscles (hip extensors) also work hard as you kick. The outer (abductor) and inner (adductor) thigh muscles are typically underused unless doing the breaststroke. If you are a swimmer, add the following exercises to either Routine A or B:

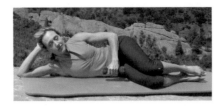

1. Rotator Cuff, page 201

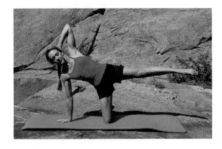

2. Kneeling Side Kicks, page 162

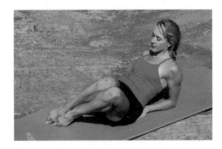

3. Cancan, page 180

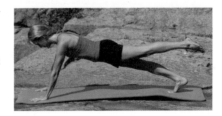

4. Leg Pull-Front, page 160

After-Training Stretches

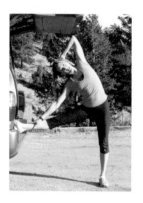

1. Two-Minute Tailgate Stretches, page 218

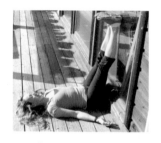

2. Wall Stretch, page 220

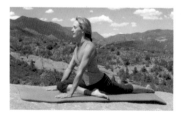

3. Pigeon Pose, page 216

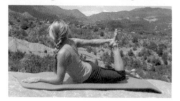

4. Quadriceps Stretch, page 217

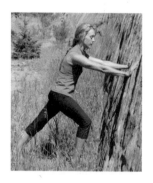

5. Calves Stretch, page 211

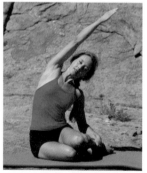

6. Mermaid, page 215

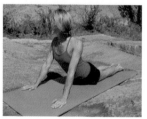

7. Neck Roll, page 216

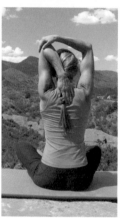

8. Triceps Stretch, page 219

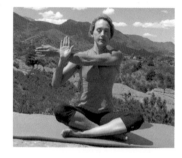

9. Shoulder Stretch, page 218

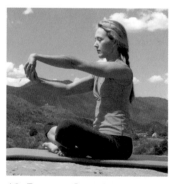

10. Forearm Stretch, page 213

Multisport

125

THE PILATES PRESCRIPTION: 15 MINUTES A DAY

Pilates in Action:
Six Tips for Multisport Athletes

To maximize the crossover of your skills from the mat to your training, here are six exercises designed to integrate your skills. Experiment with each one separately and keep them in mind as a checklist for enhancing the efficiency of your training.

1. **Breathing:** Breathe deeply. Practice inhaling deeply and exhaling air completely, drawing in your core tightly. Create a rhythm of breathing that you can maintain throughout your workouts. Once you've been successful maintaining a pattern, change it and experiment with new ones.

2. **Centering:** Engage your core while swimming by drawing your navel up to your spine. Pretend your cycling shorts have a zipper and hold your abdomen in firmly. When you run, if you tend to sway or arch your lower back, gently tuck your tailbone toward your navel.

3. **Concentration:** Strengthen your mind-body connection. Practice your sport in a style that is focused on solving the task at hand. For example, while swimming, choose one technique you would like to improve and work on refining it during a training swim.

4. **Control:** Focus being efficient in your movements and energy expenditure.

5. **Precision:** The more attention you pay to the precision of your moves, the more aligned and energy efficient your movement will be.

6. **Flowing Motion:** As you train, create a sense of continuous effort so there is no beginning or end. You'll work your legs more uniformly, thereby reducing fatigue and muscle imbalances.

Chapter 13

Joe's Mat Work

This chapter includes 32 original Pilates mat exercises from Joseph Pilates' book, *Return to Life*. Each exercise description comes complete with the following information:

1. Purpose of the Exercise

2. Level of Difficulty

3. Number of Repetitions

4. Exercise Description

5. Modifications

Purpose of the Exercise

Pilates exercises work many muscles simultaneously. Some muscles are strengthened while others are stretched. Depending on your specific strengths and weaknesses, the exercise may more effectively target one muscle group for you than it does for someone else. Keep in mind that when done properly, all Pilates exercises engage your core.

Level of Difficulty

The exercises have been categorized as beginner, intermediate, or advanced. The difficulty level is based the requirements for strength, flexibility, core strength, balance, and coordination. Because Pilates exercises build on one another, you'll want to master the easier exercises before moving on to the more challenging ones.

Number of Repetitions

Only do the recommended number of repetitions. Avoid going gang-busters and doing 100 of anything (with the exception of the Hundred). Respect and trust the method. It's worked for thousands of athletes all over the world; it can work for you, too. The work doesn't become more challenging by doing more reps; it becomes more challenging by perfecting your form. Just as in sports, there are many techniques you can improve upon. Higher-quality movement means expending less energy and reducing wear and tear on your joints. Do 50 repetitions of any exercise and your form will be sloppy and your mind will wander. Remember that Pilates is first and foremost movement training. If you want more of a workout, add more exercises. Refer to Appendix A in the back of the book to select exercises that suit your cross-training needs.

Exercise Description

Each description is accompanied by a sequence of pictures. The descriptions are concise and highlight the most important components of the exercise. Breathing cues, sequence of movement, and helpful imagery are provided. For some exercises, arrows are drawn to indicate flow of movement, accentuate key details, and highlight pitfalls.

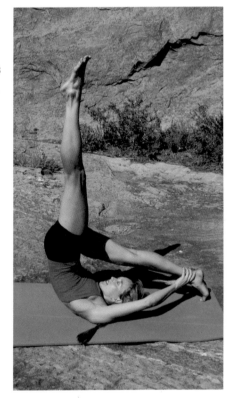

Modifications

The human body is a fabulously complex machine. When teamed with a willing mind and passionate spirit, it has the power to scale cliffs, finesse rivers, navigate mountain slopes, and the endurance to race alongside the wind. If you want to enjoy the journey and not get stranded, pay close attention to what your body is telling you. A healthy body is resilient, moves with ease, and lasts a lifetime. But it can't do this without a mind attentive to its needs. Continuously pushing the body too far is like redlining an engine. Eventually something will be damaged. Know your body and be realistic in your expectations. Caring for your body means honoring its limitations.

Many athletes have conditioned themselves to push through pain and pride themselves on having a high tolerance for pain. Pilates is different—pain equals no gain.

Experiencing pain in your lower back, shoulders, or any other joint is a red flag. Either you are doing the exercise wrong or your body is trying to tell you something and you should pay attention. Be aware of seemingly unrelated aches or pains. For example, a nervy pain running down the side of your leg can be caused by a herniated disc.

The body is very good at communicating when something is wrong. It s your job to listen. If a Pilates exercise hurts or causes discomfort, you may be doing it incorrectly. Consider modifying the exercise or omitting it altogether. The most common exercise modifications are listed for easy reference. For a complete guideline on modifications, please refer to Appendix E under "Modifications." There, you will also find tips for making exercises more challenging.

The Hundred

PURPOSE	DIFFICULTY	REPS
Warms up the circulatory system and prepares the heart for work. Strengthens the abdominal muscles and triceps.	Beginner	100 pulses

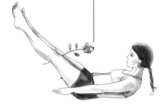

1. Begin by lying on your back with your knees bent to your chest and your arms by your side. Pull your navel to your spine. INHALE, lift your head, and curl up to your shoulder blades. Extend your arms by your sides and EXHALE, straightening your legs out to a 45-degree angle. Pull your stomach tight as a drumhead. Squeeze your legs together as if holding a rose between your knees. Breathe deeply as if to smell it.

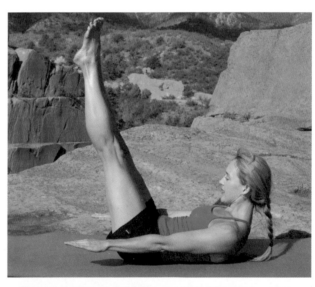

2. Pump your arms by your sides as if slapping your hands on water. INHALE for five pumps, EXHALE for five pumps, keeping everything still except for your arms. Avoid arching your lower back. Avoid tensing your shoulders or holding your breath.

3. When you reach 100 pumps, bend your knees to your chest. Relax your head, neck, shoulders, and arms down on the mat.

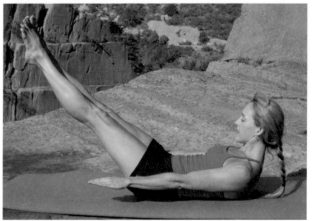

Modifications: If your lower back arches, bend your knees, bringing your legs closer to your chest, or place your feet flat on the floor. If you have had a neck injury, keep your head on the mat. If you begin to hyperventilate, try to INHALE for 3 pumps and EXHALE for 3 pumps.

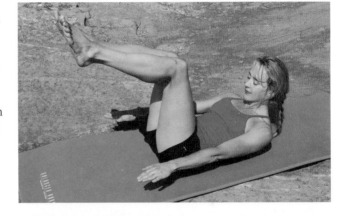

Extra Challenge: Lower your legs and work slightly lower.

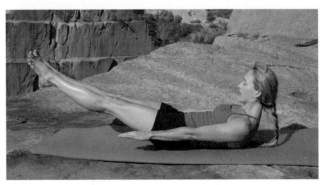

Roll Up

PURPOSE	DIFFICULTY	REPS
Strengthens the abdominal muscles.	Intermediate	6–8
Stretches the hamstrings, back, and shoulders.		
Improves spinal articulation and alignment.		

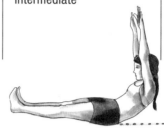

1. Begin by lying on your back with your feet flexed and your arms overhead. Pull your navel to your spine.

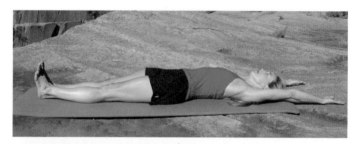

2. INHALE, raise your arms up toward the sky, and lift your head to look at your feet. Curl up, peeling your spine off the mat, as if rolling up a painting. Avoid using momentum to hoist yourself off the mat. Pretend you are under a very low sky and stay rounded throughout the exercise. Keep your heels connected to the floor as you roll up.

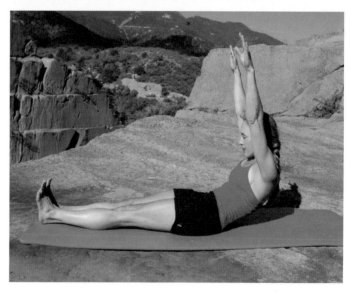

3. EXHALE and curl forward, reaching toward your feet, looking down at your knees. Hollow out your stomach as if there were something on your lap that you want to lift up over.

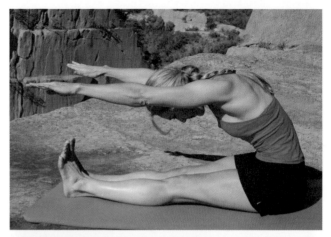

4. INHALE and roll back down one vertebra at a time, as if you were making an imprint with your spine in sand. Keep your feet flexed and imprint your spine on the mat, ending with your arms overhead. EXHALE to complete.

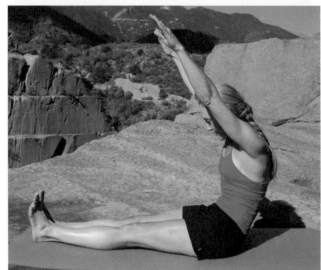

Modifications: Begin with your arms by your sides. As you begin to roll up, walk your hands up the sides of your legs. If your heels lift as you roll up, bend your knees slightly and place your feet against a wall.

Roll Over

PURPOSE	DIFFICULTY	REPS
Strengthens the abdominal muscles, shoulders, and triceps. Stretches the hamstrings and back. Improves spinal articulation.	Intermediate	3 forward, 3 in reverse

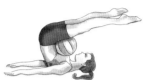

1. Begin by lying on your back with your arms by your sides, palms pressing down, legs straight up and together, toes pointed to the sky.

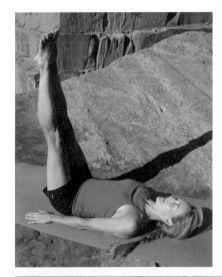

2. INHALE and peel your spine off the mat (use your core and triceps to lift, not momentum) until your legs are over your head and parallel with the floor. Imagine you have a beach ball on your lap and lift your torso up and over the ball. Avoid squashing your neck by keeping a little space between it and the mat.

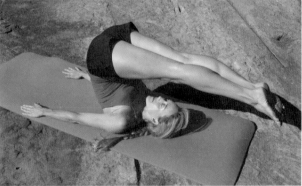

3. Open your legs the width of your mat and flex your feet.

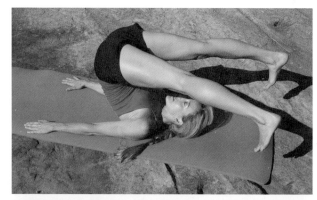

4. EXHALE and roll your spine back onto the mat to the starting position.

5. To do the exercise in reverse, begin with your legs straight up and open, toes pointed to the sky. INHALE to peel your spine off the mat until your legs are over your head and parallel with the floor. Flex your feet and bring your legs together. Exhale and roll your spine back onto the mat.

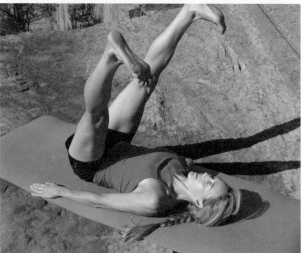

Modifications: If you have difficulty rolling up, try bending your knees to your chest and gently rock up onto your upper back and shoulders using your core. Avoid squashing your neck.

Extra Challenge: As you roll over, allow your feet to touch the floor behind you.

One-Leg Circles

PURPOSE	DIFFICULTY	REPS
Strengthens the abdominal muscles, quadriceps, and hip flexors. Stretches the hip extensors, hamstrings, and iliotibial band.	Beginner 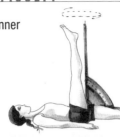	5 clockwise, 5 counter-clockwise on each leg

1. Begin by lying on your back. Extend one leg along the floor and flex your foot as if pressing it against a wall. Press the back of your leg into the floor. Extend the other leg up toward the sky and point your toes. Engage your core by pulling your navel to your spine.

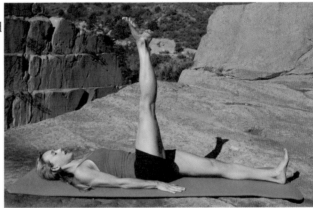

2. INHALE and sweep your raised leg horizontally across the midline of your body, down, and EXHALE up to the starting point. Keep your circle size within the borders of your mat. Although the exercise is called leg circles, imagine you are drawing ovals on the sky. Imagine your leg is connected into your belly and move your leg from your center. Keep your leg connected with your hip.

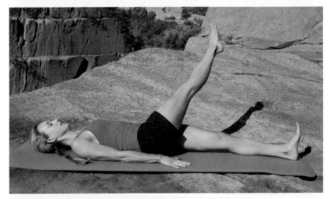

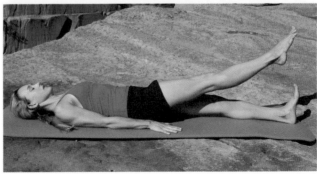

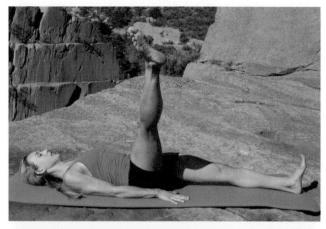

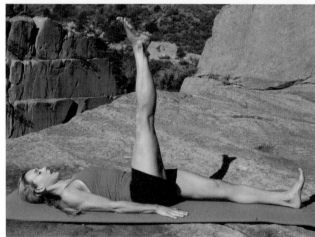

3. To reverse your circle, INHALE and sweep your leg slightly out and away from your body, then down toward the floor, and EXHALE across and back up to the starting position. Repeat five times and switch legs.

Modifications: For extra support, place the sole of your foot against a wall. For tight hip flexors or lower back, bend the outstretched leg and place the sole of your foot on the floor. If you experience hip clicking, experiment with turning your leg out to eliminate the clicking. If you experience any pain or discomfort in your hips, omit the exercise.

Rolling Like a Ball

PURPOSE	DIFFICULTY	REPS
Strengthens the abdominal muscles. Stretches the back. Improves spinal articulation.	Beginner 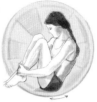	6

1. From a seated position, bend your knees and place your hands on your ankles. Bring the inside border of your feet together and your knees shoulder-width apart. Bring your heels close to your sitz bones and your shoulders down. Lift your feet off the mat and balance on the flat part of your lower spine. Gaze at your belly and keep your chin close to your chest. Pretend you are holding a nectarine under your chin and must avoid dropping it throughout the exercise. Pull your navel to your spine and gently tuck in your tailbone, stretching your lower back.

2. INHALE and tip backwards, rolling onto your shoulders, maintaining your tight, round shape. Roll yourself like a wheel rolling on a rail. Avoid throwing your head back or rolling onto your neck.

3. EXHALE and roll back up to your starting position. Avoid using momentum or bouncing through your spine.

Modifications: If you bounce through your spine or have difficulty rolling back up, bring your knees together and scoop up your legs with your arms under your thighs, grabbing your elbows. Roll as before. Padding the floor with extra mats or a blanket makes rolling more comfortable. For more challenge, wrap your arms around the outside of your lower legs and grab your elbows. Tuck your head and gaze down at your stomach.

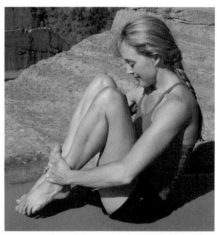

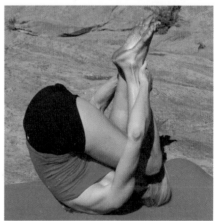

One-Leg Stretch

PURPOSE	DIFFICULTY	REPS
Strengthens the abdominal muscles.	Beginner	24
Stretches and strengthens the hip flexors.		

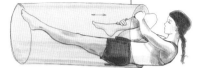

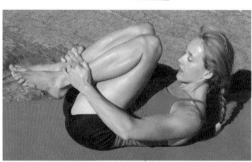

1. Begin by lying on your back, hugging your knees into your chest. Lift your head and curl up to the base of your shoulder blades. Create a C-curl in your spine and look toward your belly. Extend the left leg out at a 45-degree angle. Hug the right leg close to your chest, place your right hand above your right ankle and your left hand below your kneecap. This will enable you to pull your knee directly to your chest without twisting your leg.

2. Use a two-count INHALE, extending one leg while hugging the other knee to the chest. Switch.

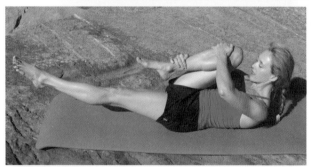

3. Use a two-count EXHALE, extending one leg while hugging the opposite knee into your chest. Imagine doing this exercise inside a cylinder and reach through the ball of your foot as if to touch the end cap. Keep your kneecaps facing the sky. Allow the inside of the legs to pass each other. Stay centered between your hips and avoid rocking side to side.

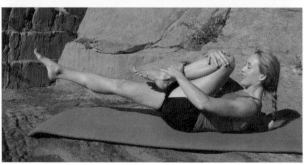

Modifications: If your lower back arches, extend your legs higher toward the sky. For more challenge, bring your legs lower, skimming your heels above the floor.

Double-Leg Stretch

PURPOSE	DIFFICULTY	REPS
Strengthens the abdominal muscles. Stretches the shoulders.	Beginner	8

1. Begin by lying on your back, hugging your knees into your chest. Lift your head and curl up to the base of your shoulder blades. Create a C-curl in your spine and look toward your belly. Pull your navel to your spine.

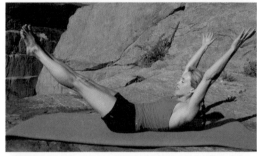

2. INHALE and reach your arms and legs out at opposite 45-degree angles. Maintain your C-curl and keep your lower back on the mat. Make yourself into the shape of a hammock. Your eyes should be on your belly, not the sky.

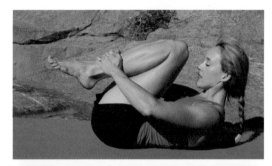

3. EXHALE, squeezing all the air out of your lungs as you sweep your arms out to the sides, and hug your knees into your chest. Make yourself tiny like a ball.

Modifications: Modify this exercise by extending your legs and arms up toward the sky. To make the exercise more challenging, extend your legs lower toward the floor. Remember to avoid arching your back.

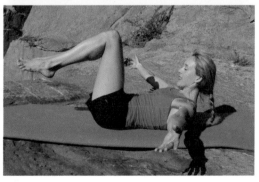

Spine Stretch

PURPOSE	DIFFICULTY	REPS
Strengthens the abdominal muscles.	Beginner	5

Stretches the hamstrings and upper back.

Improves alignment.

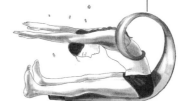

1. Sit with your legs straight out, feet slightly wider than the width of your mat. Flex your feet as if you were sitting inside a tiny sandbox and pressing your feet against the frame. Pull your navel to your spine. Pretend you have an imaginary wall behind you. Float your arms up in front of you to shoulder height and energize your arms so that all the muscles engage, as if turning on light tubes. INHALE and stretch up tall, creating a feeling of buoyancy.

2. EXHALE and curl forward from your head, bending through your spine and looking at your belly with your nose to your navel. Imagine curling into yourself like a New Year's party favor, staying lengthened out front to back, or retreating into your shell like a tiny snail. Avoid rolling your knees in or out. Do not collapse forward. Keep your shoulders relaxed.

3. INHALE and stack yourself, reinflating like a balloon. Stack your spine tall against an imaginary wall. Begin with your tailbone and articulate one vertebra at a time, until your head is on top.

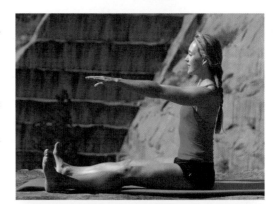

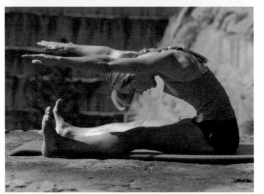

Modifications: If tight hamstrings make it difficult for you to sit up straight, roll up your mat and sit on it or sit on something (such as stacked books) so your spine will be straight.

Open-Leg Rocker

PURPOSE	DIFFICULTY	REPS
Strengthens the abdominal muscles.	Intermediate	6
Stretches the hamstrings and back.		
Improves balance.		
Lengthens the spine.		
It's a great party trick.		

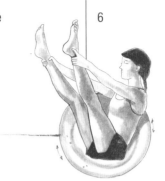

1. Beginning from a seated position, bend your knees and grab hold of the outside of your ankles. Bring the inside borders of your feet together and your knees hip-width apart. Pull your navel to your spine and lift your sternum. Maintain a roundness in your lower spine by hollowing out your belly and sitting back behind your sitz bones.

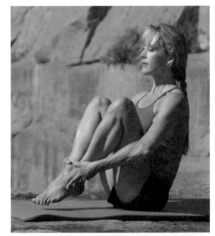

2. INHALE and stretch the right leg up. EXHALE and bend your knee, bringing your heel close to your sitz bones. Alternate, repeating 3 times on each side.

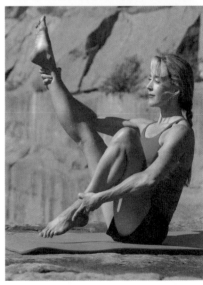

3. INHALE, lift both legs straight. EXHALE, bend your legs back to the starting position. Keep your arms connected into your shoulders and continue to lift your sternum. If this proves difficult, bend your knees to maintain better form. Repeat this step 3 times.

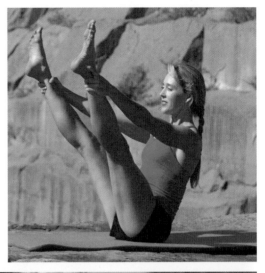

4. Lift both legs straight. Draw your navel to your spine. INHALE and roll back onto your shoulders. Keep your round shape as if you were trapped inside a giant ball. Roll onto your shoulders, not your neck. EXHALE and roll back up. Lift your sternum.

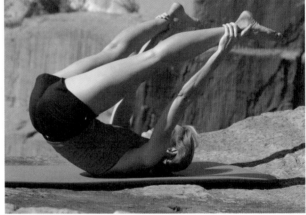

Modifications: For tight hamstrings, bend your legs slightly and hold on behind your calves instead of at the ankle. For more challenge, repeat the roll with your legs together.

Corkscrew

PURPOSE	DIFFICULTY	REPS
Strengthens the abdominal muscles, including the internal and external obliques.	Intermediate	6 each direction
Stretches the hip extensors.		

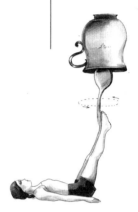

1. Begin by lying on your back with your arms by your sides, palms facing down, and legs straight up, perpendicular to your body. Zip your legs together as if they were one. Engage your core, pulling your navel to your spine.

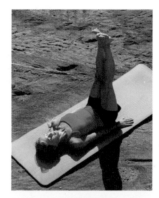

2. INHALE and circle your legs to the right, down, and up, EXHALE center. Pretend your legs are a giant spoon stirring the inside of a giant teacup that's upside down over your head and that the hand holding the spoon is your belly. Move your legs from your center. Avoid arching your back or scrunching the back of your neck. Keep your shoulders down. Switch directions each rotation.

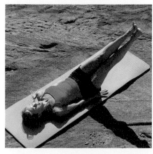
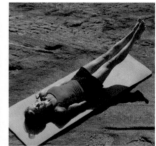

Modifications: For additional lower-back support, place your hands under your hips. You can also bend your knees and draw the circles from your kneecaps.

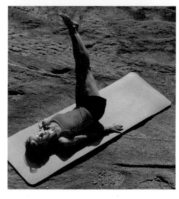

Extra Challenge: Make larger circles.

Saw

PURPOSE	DIFFICULTY	REPS
Strengthens the abdominal muscles, including the internal and external obliques.	Beginner	3 each direction

Strengthens the abdominal muscles, including the internal and external obliques.

Stretches the hamstrings and torso.

Improves alignment.

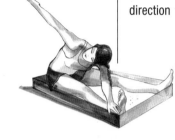

1. Sit with your feet slightly wider than the width of your mat. Pretend you are sitting inside a tiny sandbox and press the back of your hips and the bottom of your feet against the insides of the box. Reach your arms out to your sides. Energize your arms like light tubes and pretend that you intend to touch the opposite sides of the room. Avoid hyperextending your elbows. Stack your spine tall against an imaginary wall. Pull your navel to your spine.

2. INHALE and lengthen your spine, reaching up through the crown of your head as if someone were pulling you up by a string. Rotate your spine and rib cage to the right as if you were unscrewing a cylinder. Keep your arms extending from your shoulders like blades.

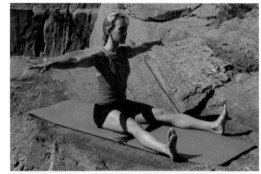

3. EXHALE and curl your spine over your right leg, sawing the pinky finger of your left hand past the right leg's pinky toe. Keep your sitz bones anchored and your kneecaps facing up instead of out or in. Avoid slumping forward over your leg. Look behind you and press the palm of the hand behind you up, as if to hold the sky up.

4. INHALE, untwist, and uncurl back up to center. EXHALE, twist, and curl to the opposite side.

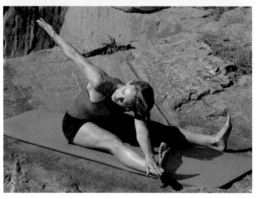

Modifications: If tight hamstrings make it difficult for you to sit up straight, roll up your mat and sit on it or sit on something (such as stacked books) so your spine will be straighter.

Swan Dive

PURPOSE	DIFFICULTY	REPS
Strengthens the back and shoulders.	Advanced	6
Stretches the abdominal muscles and hip flexors.		

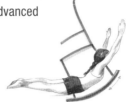

1. Begin by lying on your stomach with your palms flat, fingertips in line with your shoulders, elbows hugged in by your side, and forehead on the mat. Draw your legs tightly together. Pull your tailbone toward your belly button. Engage your core.

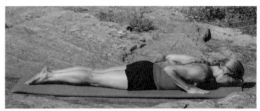

2. INHALE and gently press up through the palms of your hands, curling up, extending your spine, keeping your ribs knitted together. Pretend you are inside a ball. Lead the movement with your eyes and follow the curve of the inside of the ball with your gaze.

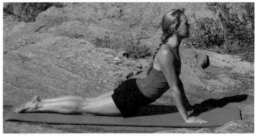

3. For the "dive," EXHALE and lift your arms straight up and out, close to your ears with palms facing in and thumbs up, and rock onto your chest and back up. Keep squeezing your legs together and pulling your navel to your spine. Make your body like the rocker of a rocking chair.

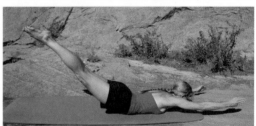

4. After six dives, catch yourself with your palms.

5. Counterpose this exercise by sitting back on your heels in Child's Pose (see page 212) to stretch your back.

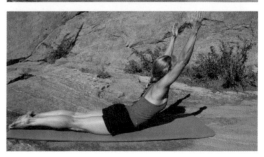

Modifications: Swan Rocking is a great way to build up to Swan Dive. Instead of reaching your arms up over your head, bend your elbows into your sides and catch yourself on your palms after each rocking. For Swan Rocking, see Chapter 14.

One-Leg Kick

PURPOSE	DIFFICULTY	REPS
Strengthens the hamstrings and hip extensors.	Beginner	6 times each leg

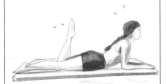

Stretches the abdominal muscles, hip flexors, and quadriceps.

Emphasizes shoulder stabilization.

1. Begin by lying on your stomach with your legs straight and together. Anchor your hip bones to the floor. Rise onto your elbows, bringing your elbows under your shoulders and your hands into fists with the knuckles pressing into each other. Pressing into your elbows and pelvic bone will help you to anchor yourself to the mat and keep your shoulder down.

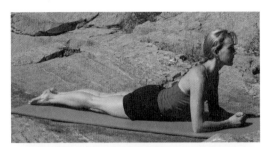

2. DOUBLE EXHALE. Bending at the knee, lift your right leg and do two half-kicks with your heel toward your bottom. Pretend you're floating on a raft in the pool. Avoid pressing your knees into the floor and stay lifted and light so the water doesn't spill onto your raft. Resist slouching into your shoulders and letting your chest cave in.

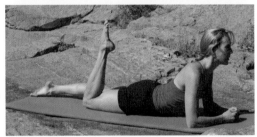

3. INHALE to extend your right leg back and down and begin two half-kicks with your left leg. Alternate.

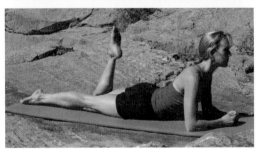

Modifications: For additional lower-back support, place a pillow under your hips and lower abdominals. If this hurts your lower back, stop and stretch out your back in Child's Pose (see page 212). If having your hands in fists is uncomfortable, place your palms flat on the mat.

Double-Leg Kick

PURPOSE	DIFFICULTY	REPS
Strengthens the hamstrings, hip extensors, and the back.	Intermediate	3–4 on each side

Stretches the chest, shoulders, and hip flexors.

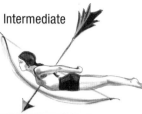

1. Begin by lying on your stomach with your head turned to one side, legs together, and hands together on the small of your back with elbows bent. If you are able to do so, bring your elbows down to the mat. Pull your tailbone toward your navel and keep your hip flexors on the mat. Zip the back of your legs together. INHALE to prepare.

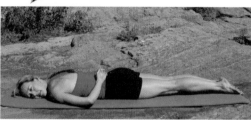

2. EXHALE. Bending at the knees, kick 3 half-kicks with your heels toward your bottom. Keep the front of your hips glued to the mat while kicking. End the last half-kick by bringing both feet onto the mat.

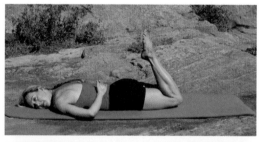

3. INHALE; roll your shoulders back and down so that your shoulder blades slide down your back. Make yourself into a bow shape and extend your spine, reaching your arms and clasped hands toward your feet. Avoid crunching up your neck.

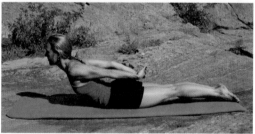

4. Switch sides by turning your head and resting the opposite cheek to the mat. Repeat.

Modifications: If you have limited range of motion in the shoulders or discomfort, bring your arms by your sides instead of behind your back. As you extend your spine, reach your fingers toward the sides of your legs as if to touch your feet.

Neck Pull

PURPOSE	DIFFICULTY	REPS
Strengthens the core. Stretches the hamstrings and back.	Intermediate 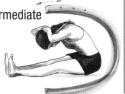	3–5

1. Begin by lying on your back with your legs straight and feet flexed hip-width apart. Bending at your elbows, support your head by stacking the palms of your hands at the base of your head, gently lengthening your neck. Draw your navel to your spine.

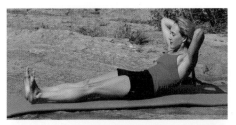

2. INHALE and lift your head to look at your feet. Peel your spine off the mat one vertebra at a time and EXHALE, curling forward as if you wanted to touch your nose to your navel. Scoop out your abdominals and avoid pulling with your arms or using momentum to hoist yourself up. Your heels should maintain contact with the floor.

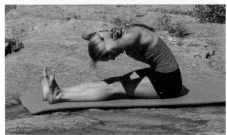

3. INHALE as you begin to stack your spine up very tall against an imaginary wall. Begin to float your torso back, hinging from your hips to the point where your heels still maintain contact with the floor.

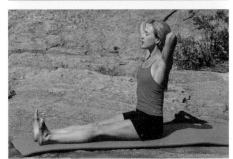

4. EXHALE; and from your tailbone begin rounding down with your spine, imprinting each vertebra onto the mat with control.

Modifications: If you find yourself pulling with your arms or having trouble not using momentum, try doing the exercise with your arms by your sides. You can walk your hands down the sides of your legs as you come up. You can also add support by placing your feet against a wall or anchoring them with a strap, couch, or ankle weights.

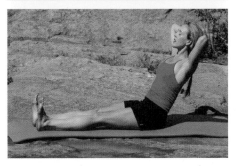

Joe's Mat Work

149

YOUR TOOLBOX

Scissors

PURPOSE	DIFFICULTY	REPS
Strengthens the abdominal muscles, shoulders, and arms.	Advanced	6

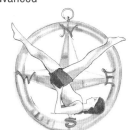

Stretches the hamstrings, quadriceps, and hip flexors.

1. Begin by lying on your back.
   Bend your knees into your chest and roll up so your weight is on your shoulders. Place your hands under your hips with your thumbs on the outside.
   Extend your legs straight up toward the sky. Make sure your weight is not on your neck.

2. INHALE; reach your legs evenly in opposite directions, front to back like hands that are connected to the center of the clock. Keep your hips lifted and level and your legs straight.

3. EXHALE; then scissor your legs past each other, reaching in opposite directions.

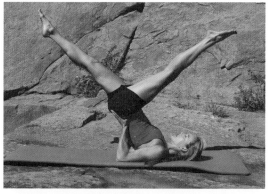

Modifications: For tight hamstrings, make the scissor movement smaller but work to reach your legs equally in both directions. If you have a wrist, elbow, or shoulder injury, consider omitting this exercise.

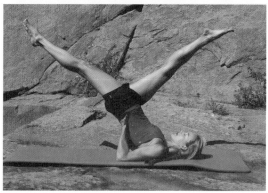

Bicycle

PURPOSE	DIFFICULTY	REPS
Strengthens the abdominal muscles, shoulders, and arms. Stretches the hamstrings, quadriceps, and hip flexors.	Advanced 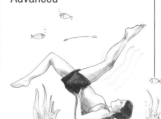	5 forward, 5 reverse

1. Begin by lying on your back. Bend your knees into your chest and roll up so your weight is on your shoulders. Place your hands under your hips with your thumbs on the outside. Extend your legs straight up toward the sky. Make sure your weight is not on your neck.

2. INHALE; bicycle your legs, reaching them evenly in opposite directions, front to back, creating a sense of resistance as if you were under water. Keep your hips lifted and level. As you straighten one leg, simultaneously bend the other leg. This will create a hamstring stretch for the straightening leg and a quadriceps stretch for the bending leg.

3. EXHALE; bicycle your legs past each other, reaching in opposite directions.

Modifications: For tight hamstrings, make the bicycle movement smaller but work to reach your legs equally in both directions. If you have a wrist, elbow, or shoulder injury, consider omitting this exercise.

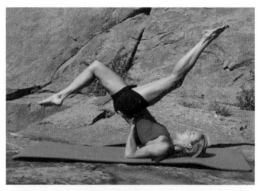

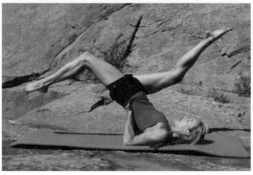

Shoulder Bridge with Kicks

PURPOSE	DIFFICULTY	REPS
Strengthens the hamstrings and back. Stretches the quadriceps and hip flexors.	Beginner 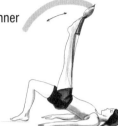	5–10 kicks with each leg

1. Lie on your back. Press your arms gently into the mat by your sides so that your chest is open and the front of your ribs recede into the mat. Bend your knees and bring your feet hip-width apart, toes pointing forward. Peel up your spine one vertebra at a time off the mat, beginning with your tailbone until you are resting on your shoulders with an open chest and an engaged core. Straighten and extend one leg and point your toes so your knees are touching.

2. INHALE, kicking up to the sky. Avoid arching your back or letting your hips tilt or lower and lift.

3. EXHALE, flex your foot, and extend the leg down, keeping it straight. Pretend your leg is a paintbrush and you are painting a straight line of your favorite color on the sky. After 5–10 kicks, repeat with the opposite leg.

Modifications: Lift your pelvis a smaller distance so you have more of your back on the mat. Omit the kicks and hold while you breathe deeply for 30 seconds to a minute.

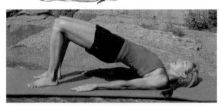
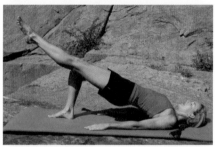
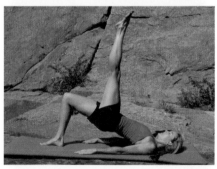
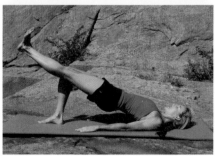

Spine Twist

PURPOSE	DIFFICULTY	REPS
Strengthens the core (internal and external obliques).	Intermediate	5 times each direction

Improves alignment and spinal rotation.

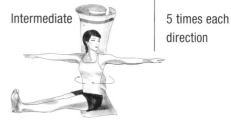

1. Begin by sitting with your legs together and out straight with your back tall as if stacked against an imaginary wall. Flex your feet as if there were a floor beneath them. Extend your arms out to your sides at shoulder height and reach through your fingers as if you intend to touch the sides of the room. Pull your navel to your spine.

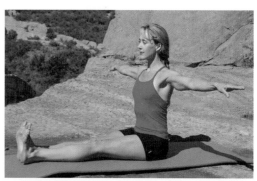

2. INHALE; lengthen up through the crown of your head as if someone were pulling you up by a string.

3. EXHALE; twist your spine. Keep your heels glued together and avoid slumping as you twist. Pretend you are a dishcloth and all the water is being wrung from you on the twist. Your arms should stay bladelike, extending straight out from your shoulders.

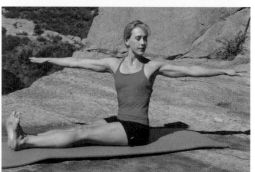

4. INHALE; lengthen your spine upward as you twist back to center. EXHALE; twist the opposite direction.

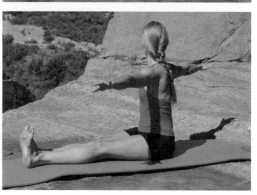

Modifications: If tight hamstrings make it difficult for you to sit up straight, roll up your mat and sit on it or sit on something (such as stacked books) to get you higher off the floor so your spine will be straighter.

Jackknife

PURPOSE	DIFFICULTY	REPS
Strengthens the abdominals and shoulders. Stretches the hamstrings and back.	Advanced	5

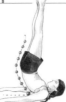

1. Begin by lying on your back with your arms by your sides, palms pressing down, backs of the arms engaged, legs straight, and toes pointed to the sky.

2. INHALE, peel your spine off the mat, and bring your legs over your head until they are parallel with the floor.

3. Lift your legs high so that they are directly above your eyes, as if being held up by a rope attached to the sky. Your weight should be balanced over your shoulders and arms.

4. EXHALE; roll your spine onto the mat one vertebra at a time, like you are placing a strand of pearls on a table.

Modifications: If you are experiencing neck or shoulder tension or your head lifts from the floor, avoid bringing your legs as high and straight over your head. Instead, allow the toes to lower behind the line of your eyes as you lift and lower down.

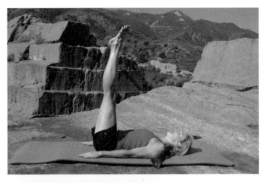

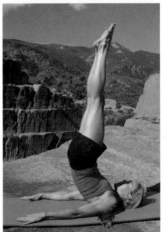

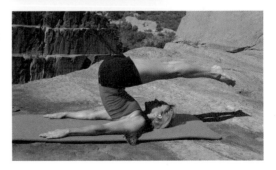

Side Kick

PURPOSE	DIFFICULTY	REPS
Strengthens the legs and hips.	Beginner	10 each side
Stretches the legs and hips.		
Improves balance and core stabilization.		

1. Begin by lying on your side. Stack your ankles, knees, hips, and shoulders. Bring your legs out on a 45-degree angle from your torso. Avoid slouching into one hip by keeping a finger's width of space under your waist. Bend the arm closest to the floor and cradle your head in your palm. Your top arm should be close in by your side with your palm pressing into the mat. Keep your shoulders down. Engage your core by pulling your navel to your spine.

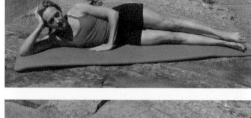

2. Lift your top leg a few inches from the bottom leg. INHALE; sweep it forward in a paintbrush-like motion using a flexed foot. Sweep the leg forward only so far as you can keep your torso still and your back from rounding. You should feel a hamstring stretch. Keep your leg straight.

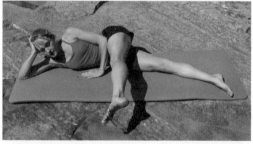

3. EXHALE; sweep the leg back with a pointed toe. Reach your leg long and away from your body to feel the hip flexor stretch.

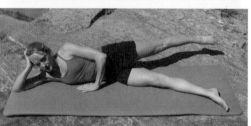

Avoid rocking your body front and back or arching your lower back. Keep your shoulders and hips perfectly still. Repeat 10 times, then switch sides.

Modifications: If you experience neck or shoulder tension, try sliding your bottom arm out straight along the mat and resting your head on your upper arm.

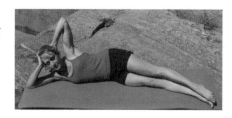

Extra Challenge: Bring your upper arm off the mat and place it behind your head.

Teaser Series

PURPOSE	DIFFICULTY	REPS
Strengthens the abdominal muscles, hip flexors, and quadriceps.	Beginner, Intermediate, or Advanced	3

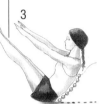

1. Lie on your back with your arms by your sides, knees bent, feet together.

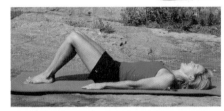

2. INHALE; curl up through your spine, floating your arms up as you come up.

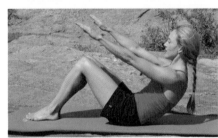

3. EXHALE to roll down your spine one vertebra at a time, floating your arms down.

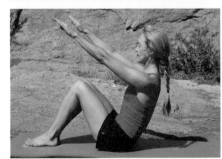

Beginner

1. Lying on your back with your legs perpendicular to your body and your toes pointed to the sky, bring your arms up over your head.

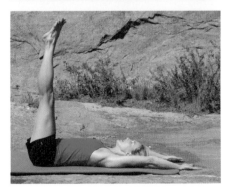

2. INHALE and curl up, tipping your torso and legs into a "V" shape. Your legs and arms should be parallel on the same diagonal.

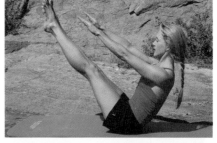

3. EXHALE, keep your legs at a 45-degree angle and roll your spine down like a strand of pearls, one pearl at a time, until you reach your shoulders. Roll back up and repeat 3 times. If you feel your back begin to arch, bend your knees and lower your feet to the floor.

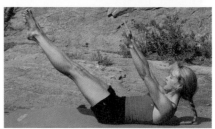

Intermediate

1. Lying on your back with your legs perpendicular to your body and your toes pointed to the sky, bring your arms up over your head.

2. INHALE and curl up, extending your legs to a 45-degree angle.

3. EXHALE and lower and lift your legs 3 times. Keep your torso at a 45-degree angle and avoid arching your back.

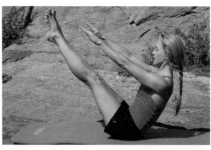

Advanced

1. Lie on your back with your arms over your head and your legs long on the floor.

2. INHALE; rolling up, lift your head and heels simultaneously while curling up into a "V" shape.

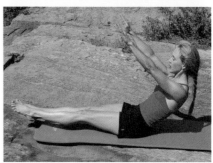

3. EXHALE and roll down your spine, lowering your legs and arms to the floor. Repeat 3 times.

Modifications: To give your lower back more support, bend your knees toward your chest.

Hip Circles

PURPOSE	DIFFICULTY	REPS
Strengthens the abdominals and hip flexors. Stretches the chest and front of the shoulders.	Advanced 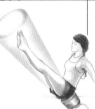	6 each direction

1. Begin by sitting on your sitz bones with your arms stretched behind you supporting your body, fingers pointed back. Your sternum is lifted, stomach firm, and legs up at a 45-degree angle.

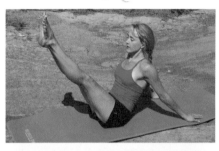

2. INHALE and begin circling your legs right, then down, then left, and EXHALE to bring the legs back up to center. Avoid arching your back and sinking into your shoulders. Pretend that your legs are like a giant light beam as you circle. Remember that the power of the light starts from the barrel that holds the light, your powerhouse.

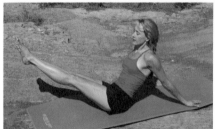

3. Reverse the circle, beginning to the left. Move left, then down and right and back to center.

Modifications: This exercise can be done by positioning yourself down on your elbows with your palms down beneath your hips.

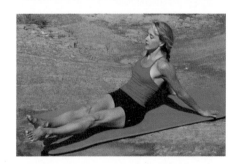

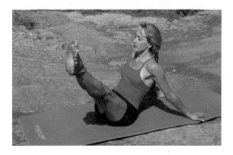

Swimming

PURPOSE	DIFFICULTY	REPS
Strengthens the back and shoulders. Stretches the abdominals and hip flexors.	Intermediate	100

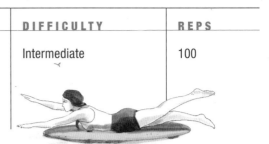

1. Lie on your stomach with your arms over your head and your legs together. Engage your core. Engage the backs of your legs and hips by zipping them together. Raise your opposite arm and leg off the floor. Simultaneously lift your head, shoulders, and sternum. Avoid scrunching up the back of your neck.

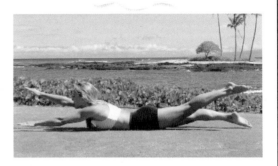

2. Paddling your arms and legs in opposition, INHALE for five counts and EXHALE for five counts. Count to 100. Pretend that you are lying on a tiny surfboard and avoid rocking side to side.

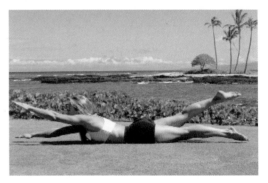

Modifications: If this exercise creates pain in the shoulders, place your arms by your sides, palms facing in, and do only the leg motion.

Joe's Mat Work

YOUR TOOLBOX

Leg Pull-Front

PURPOSE	DIFFICULTY	REPS
Strengthens the shoulders, hamstrings, and core. Stretches the calves.	Intermediate	10 on each side

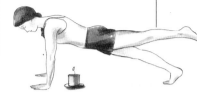

1. Begin in a push-up position, legs extended, with your hands under your shoulders and your heels over your toes. Pretend as though there were a candle under your torso and draw your abdominals in and up under your rib cage, knitting your ribs together.

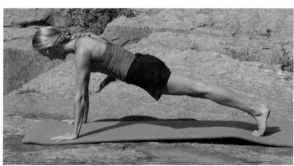

2. INHALE and lift one leg up toward the sky while pressing back through the heel of the supporting leg.

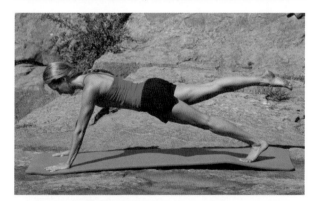

3. EXHALE, lower the leg down, and bring your opposite heel back to center.

Modifications: This exercise can also be done by supporting yourself on your elbows with the palms pressing into the floor.

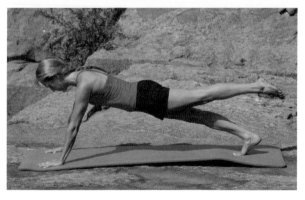

Leg Pull-Up

PURPOSE	DIFFICULTY	REPS
Strengthens the shoulders, arms, quadriceps, and hip flexors. Stretches the hamstrings, hip extensors, and chest.	Advanced 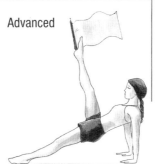	10 on each side

1. Sitting with your legs together and straight, bring your arms behind you and press up on the palms of your hands. Lift your sternum and draw your shoulders down. Gaze is forward.

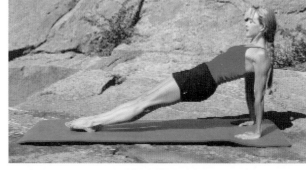

2. INHALE and kick one leg straight up like a flagpole. Avoid sinking into your shoulders or excessively rounding the spine while kicking.

3. EXHALE and place the leg down.

4. Alternate, kicking the other leg straight up.

Modifications: For wrist injuries, consider performing this exercise from the elbows.

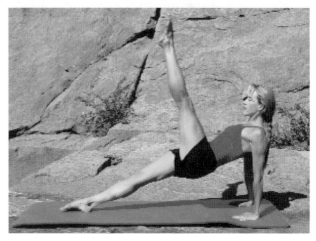

Kneeling Side Kicks

PURPOSE	DIFFICULTY	REPS
Strengthens the legs, hips, and abdominals.	Advanced	10 on each side

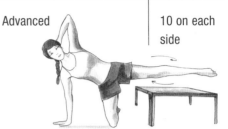

1. Begin by kneeling with your legs together and your arms reaching out to the sides at shoulder height. Tip over until you are balancing over your right arm and leg. Extend your left leg out straight. Keep your hips square and abdominals scooped. INHALE to kick the leg forward like you're kicking over a tabletop. Keep your supporting leg vertical and strong like a tree trunk.

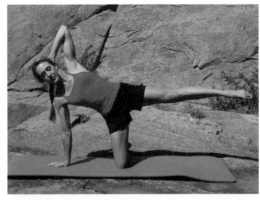

2. EXHALE to sweep the leg straight back over the imaginary tabletop. Keep your leg parallel with the floor and level with your hip.

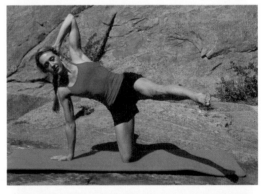

Modifications: For additional challenge, add kicking up and down and leg circles.

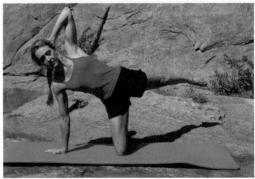

Side Bend

PURPOSE	DIFFICULTY	REPS
Strengthens the abdominals (internal and external obliques) and the shoulders.	Advanced	5

Stretches the abdominals and hips.

Improves balance.

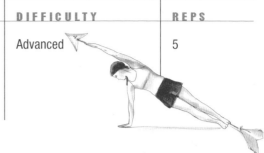

1. Sitting on one hip, extend your legs out from your torso with slightly bent knees. Place your top foot in front of your bottom foot. Rest your top arm on your leg and place your bottom arm slightly in front of your shoulder.

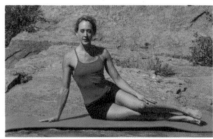

2. INHALE; press up and make yourself straight as an arrow in a side plank. Your supporting arm should be under your shoulder. Look directly forward and keep your head in line with your spine. Pretend your body is between two panes of glass.

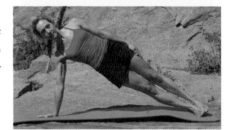

3. EXHALE; lower yourself down so you are a few inches off the ground. Avoid sinking into your shoulders or sitting down before you press back up. INHALE; raise back up and extend your top arm over your head and look at the mat. EXHALE down.

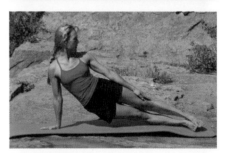

Modifications: For additional support, as you press up into your side bend, place the knee of the lower leg on the mat so that your torso is supported over your knee as you side bend.

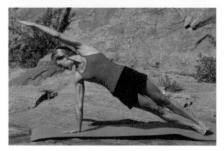

Boomerang

PURPOSE	DIFFICULTY	REPS
Strengthens your abdominal muscles.	Intermediate	6
Stretches your back, hamstrings, and shoulders.		
Improves balance.		
Improves spinal articulation.		

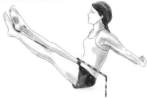

1. Begin by sitting up tall with your legs out straight, ankles crossed, and your arms by your sides.

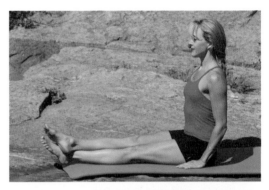

2. INHALE; roll back onto your shoulders, lifting your legs until they are parallel with the floor over your head. Avoid scrunching up your neck.

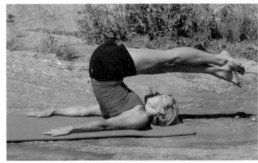

3. EXHALE; uncross and recross your legs, with the opposite ankle on top. Roll up into a Teaser "V" position (see page 157). Bring your arms out in front to the same diagonal as your legs.

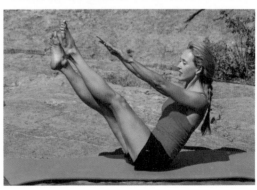

4. INHALE; sweep your arms out to your sides and behind your back. Clasp your hands, roll your shoulders back, and bring yourself forward with your head to your knees. Lift your belly up into your spine as if you are lifting over a high-jump pole.

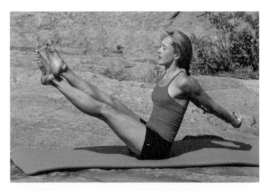

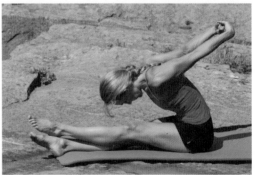

5. EXHALE; release your hands, rotate your shoulders so that your palms face the floor and stretch them out over your legs.

Modifications: For tight shoulders, do not force the hands to clasp behind the back. Instead, as you bring the arms and hands back, focus on properly rotating the shoulders.

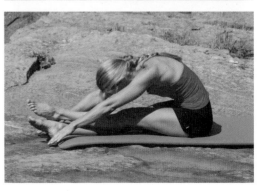

Seal

PURPOSE	DIFFICULTY	REPS
Strengthens the core. Stretches the back and hips.	Beginner 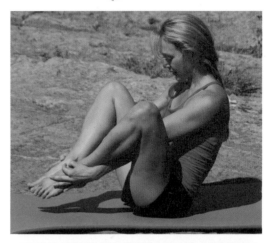	6–8

1. From a seated position, bend your knees and grapevine your hands around your legs from the inside to the outside, holding onto your ankles. Relax your hips and legs into your hands. Round your lower spine and draw your abdominals inward and upward under your rib cage. Gaze down at your belly and maintain a space the size of a nectarine between your chin and your chest.

2. Clap the inside edges of your feet together 3 times, feeling the hip flexors relax.

3. INHALE and roll back onto your shoulders, legs over your head in the same position, and clap the inside edges of your feet together 3 times. Avoid rolling onto your neck.

4. EXHALE to roll back up to start.

Modifications: If you have difficulty balancing on your shoulders, omit the back claps. As you build strength, add them in one at a time.

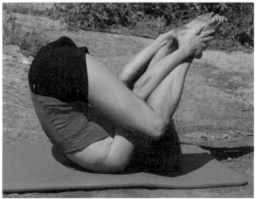

Control Balance

PURPOSE	DIFFICULTY	REPS
Strengthens the core. Stretches the hamstrings.	Advanced	10

1. Lie on your back with your legs up toward the sky and your arms overhead. Roll back onto your shoulders and extend both legs to the sky. Bring your arms overhead. Keep one leg raised as if it were tied up there by a rope, and bring the other leg down over your head and grab your ankle. Avoid smashing your neck. Your weight should be on your shoulders.

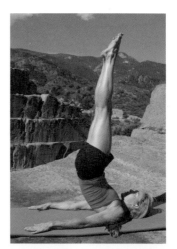

2. INHALE and alternate, scissoring your legs and grabbing hold of the opposite ankle.

3. EXHALE and alternate, scissoring your legs and grabbing hold of the opposite ankle.

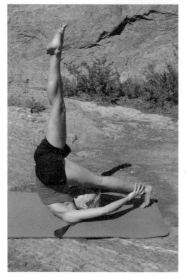
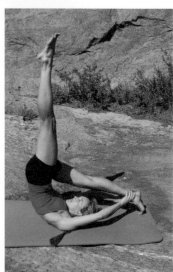

Push-Ups

PURPOSE	DIFFICULTY	REPS
Strengthen the shoulders, chest, arms, and abdominal muscles.	Intermediate	10

Stretches the hamstrings and back.

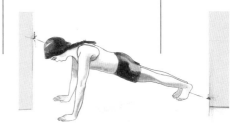

1. Begin by standing up tall with your arms over your head. Roll down one vertebra at a time until your hands are on the floor.

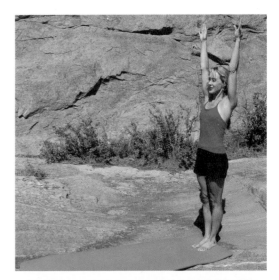

2. INHALE and walk your hands out until you are in a planklike push-up position with your arms under your shoulders. EXHALE. Pretend as though there were a rope drawn tight through your body from your head to your heels and avoid arching or rounding your spine. You should be looking directly at the floor.

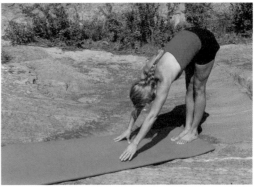

3. Use a full breath for each push-up.

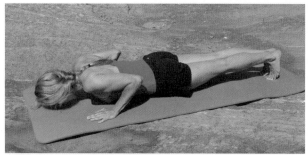

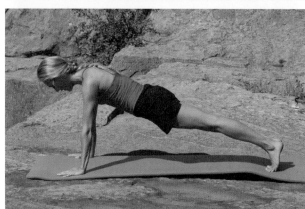

4. Walk your hands back in and roll up one vertebra at a time.

Modifications: To make the movement less strenuous, drop to the knees and do the push-ups from this position.

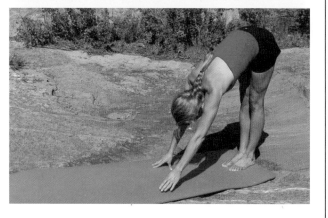

VARIATION: One-Leg Push-Ups

PURPOSE	DIFFICULTY	REPS
Strengthen the shoulders, chest, arms, and abdominal muscles. Stretches the hamstrings and back.	Intermediate	5

1. Begin by standing up tall with your arms over your head. Hinge from your hips and lift one leg behind you as you lower your torso forward and raise your leg up farther.

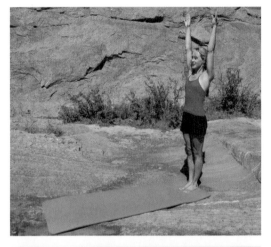

2. INHALE, keep your leg extended, and walk your hands out until you are in a planklike push-up position with your arms under your shoulders. EXHALE.

3. Use a full breath for each one-legged push-up.

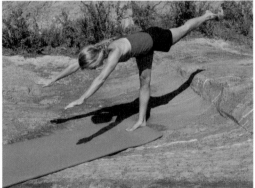

4. Walk your hands back in and lower your leg back down as you hinge back up from the hips to an upright standing position. Repeat, standing on the opposite leg.

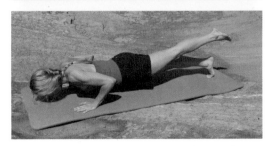

Chapter 14

Pilates Mat Maximizers

This chapter includes 31 additional Pilates exercises designed to maximize your cross-training workouts. **Exercises are arranged in three categories: lower body, core, and upper body.** Some are considered part of the original mat work developed by Joseph Pilates. Others have been adapted from the studio apparatus work, and a few gems have evolved throughout the years. Any exercise requiring or benefiting from the use of a small ball, light two- to five-pound dumbbells, or one- to two-pound ankle weights is noted.

LOWER BODY Side Kicks (8 VARIATIONS) ANKLE WEIGHTS OPTIONAL

PURPOSE	DIFFICULTY	REPS
Strengthen the legs and hip muscles.	Intermediate	10 of each on each side (except for Heel Clicks)
Stretches the hips.		
Improves core stabilization.		

Joe's original Side Kicks in Chapter 13 and the following eight variations make up the Side-Kick Series.

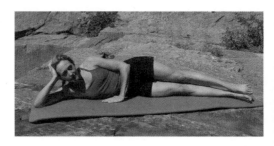

(1) Side Kicks—Paintbrush

1. Begin by lying on your side. Bend your bottom arm and rest your head on your hand. Bend your top arm and bring it close to your side, pressing your palm onto the mat. Stack your ankles, knees, hips, and shoulders. Bring your legs out on a 45-degree angle from your torso. Avoid shortening your waistline by keeping a finger's width of space under your waist and your heels stacked. Engage your core by pulling your navel to your spine.

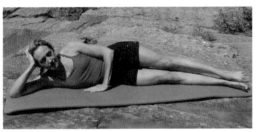

Lift your top leg about one foot from the bottom leg and slightly rotate out your leg from your hip.

2. INHALE; sweep your leg forward, keeping your torso still and your belly drawn in. You should feel a hamstring stretch.

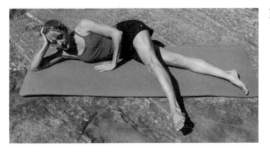

3. EXHALE; point your foot and sweep your leg back, again keeping your torso still. You should feel the hip flexor stretch. Avoid rocking your body front and back or arching or rounding your spine. Keep your shoulders and hips perfectly still.

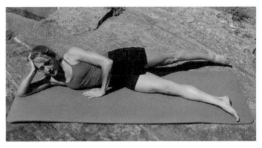

Modifications: If you have difficulty keeping your torso still, make the arc smaller.

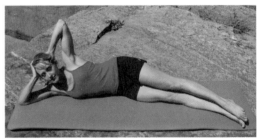

Extra Challenge: Remove your upper arm from the mat and place your hand behind your head.

(2) Side Kicks—Kick-Ups

1. Begin by lying on your side. Bend your bottom arm and rest your head on your hand. Bend your top arm and bring it close to your side, pressing your palm onto the mat. Stack your ankles, knees, hips, and shoulders. Bring your legs out on a 45-degree angle from your torso. Lengthen your waist and keep a finger's width of space under your waist. Engage your core by pulling your navel to your spine.

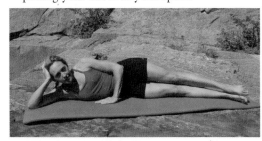

2. Externally rotate your top leg so that the top of your foot and kneecap are turned out. Keep your hips stacked.

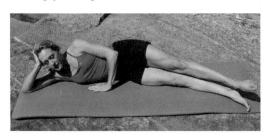

3. INHALE; kick your leg straight up toward the sky. Keep your leg straight. You should feel a hamstring stretch.

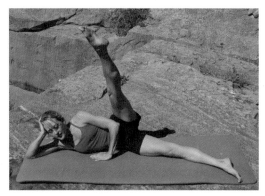

4. EXHALE and press your leg down, lengthening it away from your hip until your ankles touch. Create imaginary resistance as if you were squeezing an accordion between your legs.

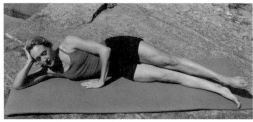

Modifications: If you have difficulty keeping your torso still, make the kick smaller.

Extra Challenge: Remove your upper arm from the mat and place your hand behind your head.

(3) Side Kicks—Circles

1. Begin by lying on your side. Bend your bottom arm and rest your head on your hand. Bend your top arm and bring it close to your side, pressing your palm onto the mat. Stack your ankles, knees, hips, and shoulders. Bring your legs out on a 45-degree angle from your torso. Lengthen both sides of your waistline and keep a finger's width of space under your waist. Engage your core by pulling your navel to your spine.

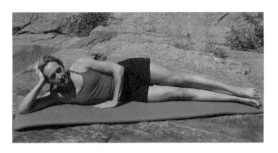

2. INHALE and begin drawing a circle with your leg. Point your toes and draw a circle the size of a pizza perpendicular to the floor.

3. EXHALE and press your leg down until your ankles touch.

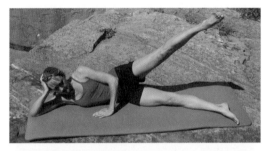

Modifications: If you have difficulty keeping your torso still, make your circles smaller.

Extra Challenge: Remove your upper arm from the mat and place your hand behind your head.

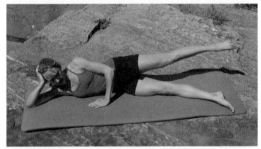

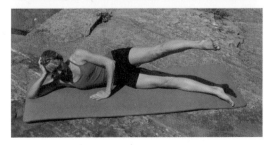

(4) Side Kicks—Lower-Leg Lifts

1. Begin by lying on your side. Bend your bottom arm and rest your head on your hand. Bend your top arm and bring it close to your side, pressing your palm onto the mat. Stack your ankles, knees, hips, and shoulders. Lift your top leg one to two feet up.

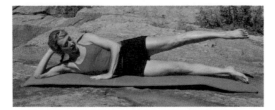

2. INHALE and lift your bottom leg up to meet your top leg. Pretend your legs are like magnetic strips that snap together as they meet. Avoid rolling back on your hips or shortening your waist as you lift.

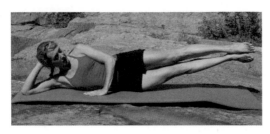

3. EXHALE and lower your leg down until it is just a few inches off the floor.

Extra Challenge: Lower your top leg to meet your bottom leg. INHALE and lift both legs together. EXHALE to lower.

(5) Side Kicks—Inner Thigh

1. Begin by lying on your side. Bend your bottom arm and rest your head on your hand. Bend your top arm and bring it close to your side, pressing your palm onto the mat. Stack your ankles, knees, hips, and shoulders. Bend your top leg, place the sole of your foot near your front hip and grab hold from the inside. Flex the outstretched foot, engaging the inner quadriceps muscles. Lengthen out your waistline and keep a finger's width of space under your waist. Engage your core by pulling your navel to your spine.

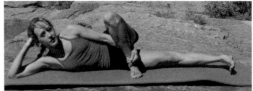

2. INHALE and lift your bottom leg up.Create resistance as you press your lower leg up by pretending you have a ski boot on your foot.

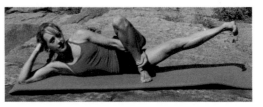

3. EXHALE and lower your leg down without touching the floor, as if your leg were buoyant.

Modifications: If you have difficulty keeping your top foot on the mat, bend your knee and rest your top leg on the mat in front of you. Remember to keep your hips stacked.

(6) Side Kicks—Scissors

1. Begin by lying on your side. Bend your bottom arm and rest your head on your hand. Bend your top arm and bring it close to your side, pressing your palm onto the mat. Stack your ankles, knees, hips, and shoulders. Lengthen both sides of your waistline and keep a finger's width of space under your waist. Engage your core by pulling your navel to your spine.

2. INHALE. Lifting your legs six inches from the floor, scissor them in opposite directions away from the midline of your body. EXHALE and scissor them past each other again. Keep your torso still as you reach your legs long and away from your hips.

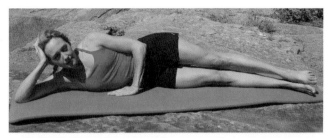

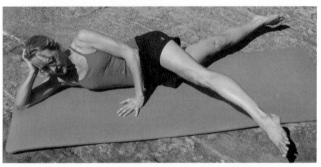

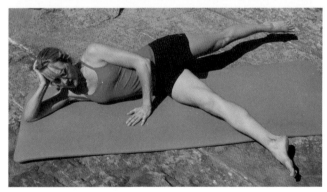

(7) Side Kicks—Bicycle

1. Begin by lying on your side. Bend your bottom arm and rest your head on your hand. Bend your top arm and bring it close to your side, pressing your palm onto the mat. Stack your ankles, knees, hips, and shoulders. Lengthen out both sides of your waistline and keep a finger's width of space under your waist.

2. INHALE, bend your top leg, grab your ankle, and pull your knee to your chest. Keep your spine straight, your chest open, and your shoulders down.

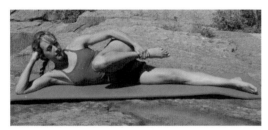

3. EXHALE, reverse your handgrip to the back side of your ankle, and extend your leg straight in front of your face. If your spine starts to bend, reduce your range of motion.

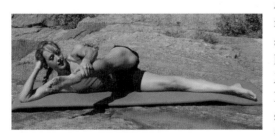

4. INHALE and release your leg, circling downward until your leg is parallel with your body. As you release, circle your arm away from your leg and over your head. Keep your hips stacked, core engaged, and torso still.

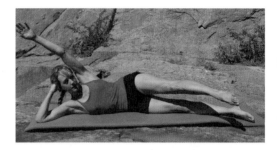

5. EXHALE; bend your knee and grab hold of your ankle. Continue to maintain a straight spine by pulling your navel to your spine. Repeat by bringing your knee to your chest.

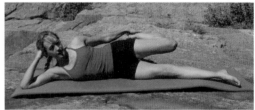

Modifications: If you have tight hamstrings, it is more important to keep your spine straight and your hips stacked than it is to be able to hold your ankle and straighten your leg. Maintain your alignment first and foremost. If you have limited range of motion in your shoulders, modify your arm circle to where it feels comfortable.

(8) Side Kicks—Heel Clicks

1. Lying on your stomach, place your hands under your forehead and bring your feet into a "V" with your heels together. Engage your core and lift your kneecaps a few inches off the floor. Zip the backs of your legs together, engaging your hamstrings and hips.

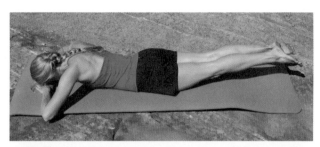

2. Click your heels together fast and furiously, keeping your legs straight. INHALE for five counts and EXHALE for five counts. Click as many times as you can in 10 seconds.

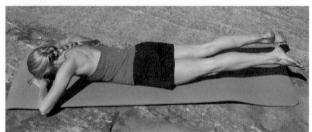

Modifications: For additional lower-back support, cup your hip bones with your hands to do the clicks.

Extra Challenge: Bend your knees and press your feet toward the sky before beginning your clicks.

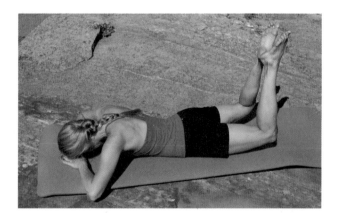

LOWER BODY Side Lunges **DUMBBELLS**

PURPOSE	DIFFICULTY	REPS
Strengthen the legs and hips.	Beginner	10 on each side
Stretches the hip flexors.		
Improves core stabilization.		

1. Begin by standing with your feet together, left foot forward, right foot turned out on a 45-degree angle, heels together, and arms by your sides.

2. INHALE, lengthen out your waistline, grow tall out of the crown of your head.

3. EXHALE; lunge out to the right side and raise your arms up to the height of your shoulders. Your right knee should be over your ankle, and you should be able to look down and see your big toe.

4. Using a full breath, lower and lift your arms 3 times before returning to center. Alternate to the left side.

Modifications: If you have a shoulder injury, omit or lighten the weight of the dumbbells.

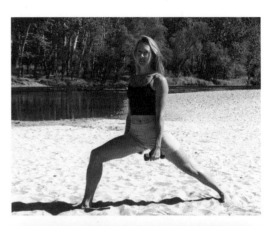

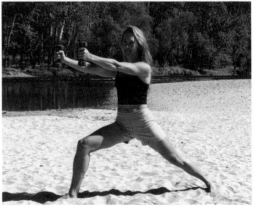

PURPOSE	DIFFICULTY	REPS
Strengthens the abdominal muscles and hip flexors. Stretches the hip extensors.	Intermediate	4–6 kicks in each direction

1. Begin by sitting on your sitz bones with your knees together and bent, your heels close to your sitz bones. Lean back, supporting your weight on your elbows. Lift your sternum and bring your shoulders down and back. Draw your navel to your spine. Lift your feet off the floor and keep the inside edges together.

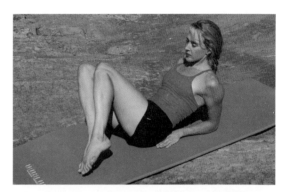

2. Swivel your hips to the right, then left, then right, and kick your legs straight, toward 2 o'clock. As you swivel, keep your knees within the frame of your body. INHALE to swivel each direction; EXHALE to kick.

3. Alternate. Swivel your hips to the left, then right, then left, and kick your legs straight, toward 10 o'clock.

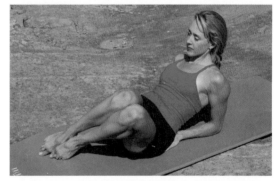

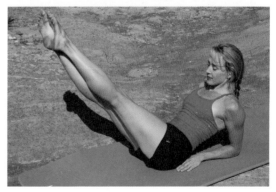

CORE Captain Crunch BALL OPTIONAL

PURPOSE	DIFFICULTY	REPS
Strengthens the abdominal muscles.	Intermediate	10
Stretches the hamstrings.		

1. Begin by lying on your back with the left leg extended along the mat and the right leg straight up to the sky. Square your hips so that both sides of your waistline are lengthened out. Bring your arms over your head. Engage your core by drawing your navel to your spine.

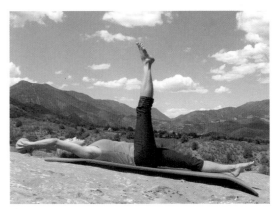

2. INHALE to prepare. EXHALE and simultaneously curl up your torso and reach your hands to touch the ankle of your left leg as it scissors up. Stretch your waistline like saltwater taffy, maximizing the distance between your hips and ribs. As you curl back down, scissor your left leg down and your right leg back up toward the sky. You may use a small ball to touch your ankles to make this exercise more interesting, but it is not required.

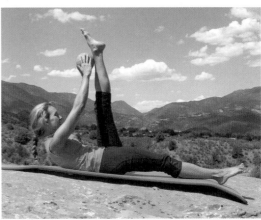

PURPOSE	DIFFICULTY	REPS
Strengthens the abdominal muscles and arms (triceps).	Intermediate	5

1. Begin by lying on your back, with your arms hugged into your sides, your knees in a tabletop position. Curl up to the base of your shoulder blades so that your gaze is at your stomach. Bend your elbows so that your fingers are pointed up towards the sky, but keep your elbows close by your sides. Engage your core and draw your navel to your spine.

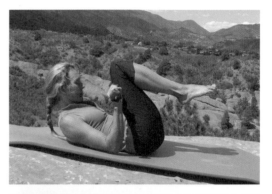

2. INHALE, extend your arms straight so that your triceps engage, and straighten your legs to a 45-degree angle. Fold your ribs into your spine and scoop your abdominals so that your lower back doesn't arch. Open and close your legs 3 times.

3. EXHALE, bend your knees into your chest, then bend your elbows so your arms come back to the 90-degree angle. Maintain your C-curl throughout the exercise.

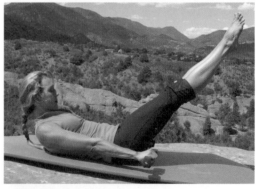

Modifications: If this causes tension in your neck or shoulders, place your head down between sets. If your back arches, keep your legs higher toward the sky.

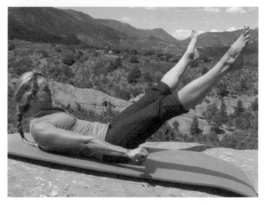

CORE Crisscross

PURPOSE	DIFFICULTY	REPS
Strengthens the abdominal muscles (internal and external obliques). Stretches the torso and shoulders. Improves spinal rotation.	Intermediate	16

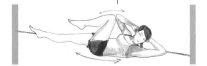

1. Begin by lying on your back with your hands stacked behind your head, elbows bent, and your knees to your chest. Curl up to the base of your shoulder blades, creating a C-curl in your spine, and look toward your belly. Maintain this C-curl shape throughout the entire exercise.

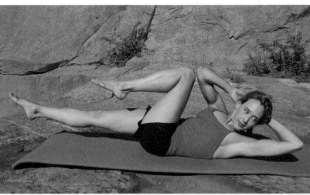

2. INHALE, rotate your rib cage, and bring your right elbow to your left knee, stretching out the right leg. Pretend you are in a cylinder and rotate within the frame of your body; avoid side bending at the waist. As you stretch one leg, pretend you are trying to touch something with your toes. Look back toward your opposite elbow as you twist, keeping your shoulders off the mat. Avoid pulling on your neck or rocking side to side. Alternate to the opposite side, keeping your legs parallel as they pass each other, kneecaps facing the sky. INHALE for one right-and-left twist, then EXHALE for one right-and-left twist.

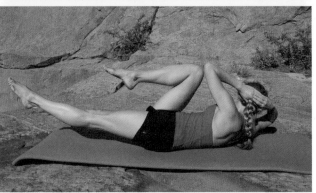

Modifications: If your lower back arches, bring your legs higher and stretch them toward the sky. For more challenge, bring legs lower, keeping heels just above the floor.

Mat Maximizers

183

YOUR TOOLBOX

PURPOSE	DIFFICULTY	REPS
Strengthens the abdominal muscles. Stretches the hamstrings.	Advanced	16

1. This Pilates exercise is an original Richard Rossiter core buster that delivers much bang for the buck. Begin by lying on your back with your knees into your chest. Lift your head, neck, and shoulders and curl up into a C-curl. Extend your arms and legs out in opposite directions at 45-degree angles. Engage your core. Avoid arching your back and draw your navel to your spine. If your back arches, bring your legs up higher.

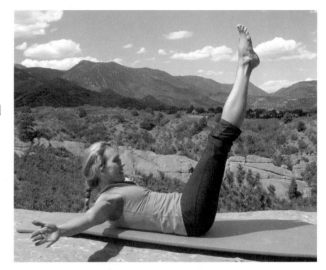

2. INHALE to prepare. EXHALE; scissor your legs lengthwise and rotate your torso so you can touch your elbow to your opposite knee.

3. INHALE and come back to center so that your legs are back at the starting position.

4. EXHALE; scissor your legs, and rotate your torso to the other side, touching the opposite elbow to your knee.

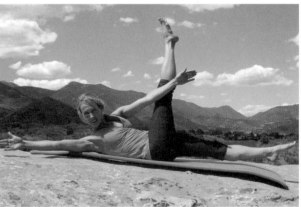

CORE Double-Straight-Leg Stretch BALL OPTIONAL

PURPOSE	DIFFICULTY	REPS
Strengthens the core.	Intermediate	6

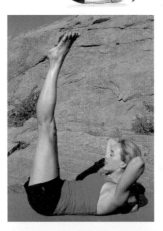

1. Begin by lying on your back. Stack your hands behind your head with your elbows bent and gently lengthen the back of your neck. Create a C-curl, rolling up to the base of your shoulder blades. Gaze at your belly and maintain your C-curl position throughout the exercise. Bring your legs perpendicular to your body. Slightly externally rotate your legs so your heels are touching and zip the backs of your thighs together.

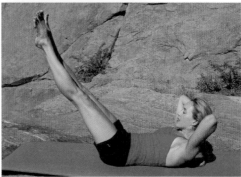

2. INHALE and lower your legs to 45 degrees. Imagine your legs are straight and solid like a door and your hips are like a hinge. Your torso should be as solid as a strong wall. Avoid arching your lower back. Keep your spine flat on the mat.

3. EXHALE and lift your legs back to perpendicular, keeping your tailbone on the mat. Only lower your legs as far as you can while still keeping your lower back on the mat.

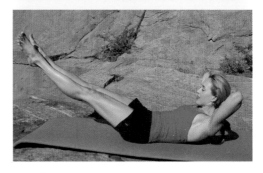

Modifications: If your lower back begins to arch away from the mat, reduce the angle at which you lower your legs.

Extra Challenge: Place a small ball between your ankles.

PURPOSE	DIFFICULTY	REPS
Strengthens the core and arms.	Intermediate	3 forward, 3 reverse

1. Begin by lying on your back, your knees to your chest. Create a C-curl, rolling up to the base of your shoulder blades so that your gaze is at your stomach. Maintain your C-curl position throughout the entire exercise. Bend your arms, make fists, and bring your hands together, knuckles touching, approximately six inches above your forehead so your arms make a circle.

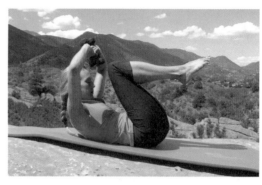

2. INHALE; extend your arms and legs straight up.

3. EXHALE; open both your arms and legs into a "V."

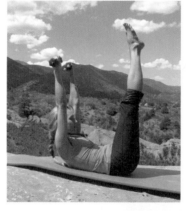
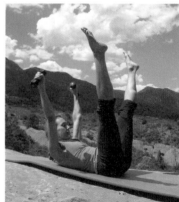

4. INHALE; circle your arms and legs down to a 45-degree angle. If your back arches, keep your legs higher.

5. EXHALE; bring your knees into your chest and your arms back to the starting position.

Modifications: To modify this exercise, omit the use of dumbbells and keep your legs higher. Make certain that your lower back does not arch.

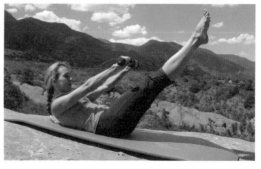

CORE Footwork

PURPOSE	DIFFICULTY	REPS
Strengthens your abdominal muscles and inner thighs.	Intermediate	10

1. Begin by lying on your back, elbows bent, with your hands stacked behind your head, and lengthen out the back of your neck. Bring your knees toward your shoulders. Lift your head, neck, and shoulders and curl up to the base of your shoulder blades, creating a C-curl shape in your upper spine. Gaze at your stomach. Maintain this C-shape throughout the entire exercise. Externally rotate your hips so that your knees are shoulder-width apart and your feet are in a "V" with the heels touching.

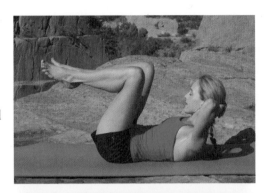

2. INHALE and extend your legs straight while keeping your heels together. Your knees should be slightly rotated outward. Create resistance by imagining that you are pushing a stack of heavy books out over an imaginary tabletop. Make sure that your lower back doesn't arch away from the floor and that your abdominals stay scooped.

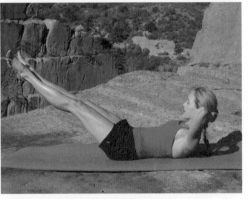

3. EXHALE and pull your feet back over the imaginary tabletop, bending the knees to the starting position.

4. Finish the series by extending legs and flexing the feet. INHALE to point. EXHALE to flex.

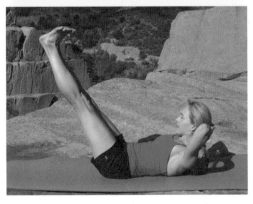

Modifications: To modify footwork, extend your legs out on a 45-degree angle as if you were sliding your heels up and down a slope.

CORE One-Straight-Leg Stretch

PURPOSE	DIFFICULTY	REPS
Strengthens the abdominal muscles. Stretches the hamstrings and hip flexors.	Beginner	10 times on each leg

1. Begin by lying on your back, hugging your knees into your chest. Lift your head, neck, and shoulders and curl up to the base of your shoulder blades, creating a C-curl shape in your upper spine. Gaze at your stomach. Maintain this C-shape throughout the entire exercise. Extend one leg out, parallel to the floor, and extend the other leg up to the sky with your hands behind your calf.

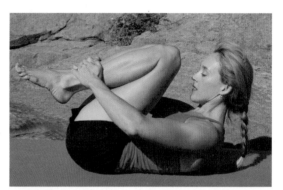

2. INHALE twice and gently pulse your raised leg twice, pulling it toward your ear.

3. Scissor your legs parallel past each other like the hands of a clock. EXHALE twice and pulse your leg twice, pulling it toward your ear. Avoid rocking side to side. Avoid hunching your shoulders up around your ears.

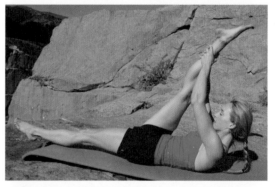

Modifications: For tight hamstrings, reach behind the thigh instead of behind the calf.

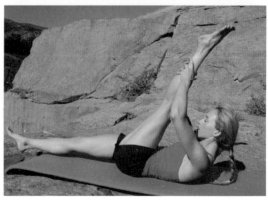

CORE Skydiver

PURPOSE	DIFFICULTY	REPS
Strengthens the back and muscles along the spine.	Intermediate	5–10

1. Lie on your stomach with your arms stretched over your head. Draw your stomach tight. Engage the backs of your legs.

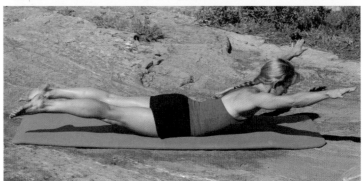

2. INHALE; lift your sternum and hover both your arms and legs off the floor.

3. EXHALE; lower yourself back down to the mat.

PURPOSE	DIFFICULTY	REPS
Strengthens the back and muscles along the spine. Stretches the chest and the front of the shoulders. Improves balance.	Advanced	3–5 on each side

1. This exercise has been adapted from the Pilates reformer. Sitting on one hip, extend your legs out long with your top foot in front of your bottom foot.

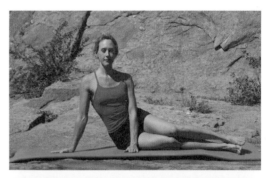

2. INHALE and rotate the back of your hips up toward the sky so your arms and legs are straight and you are on your toes.

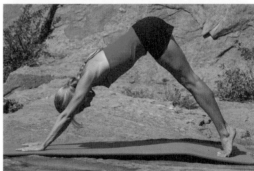

3. EXHALE and extend through your spine. Lift your sternum and draw your shoulders down, and knit your ribs together.

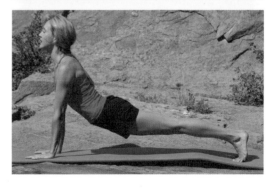

CORE Swan Rocking

PURPOSE	DIFFICULTY	REPS
Strengthens the back and shoulders.	Intermediate	6
Stretches the abdominal muscles and hip flexors.		

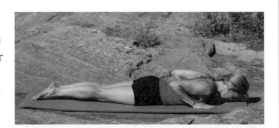

1. Begin by lying on your stomach with your palms flat on the floor, fingertips in line with your shoulders, and elbows tucked in by your sides. Draw your legs tightly together. Pull your tailbone toward your belly button. Engage your core.

2. INHALE and gently press up through the palms of your hands, curling up, extending your spine. Lift your sternum, draw your shoulders down and back, and keep your ribs knitted together. Lengthen the back of your neck.

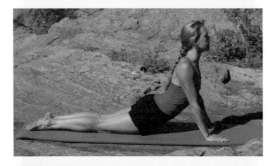

3. For the "rocking," EXHALE, bend your elbows into your sides, and rock onto your chest in a seesaw-like motion that brings your legs upward. As your torso rocks back up, catch yourself on your palms. Throughout the exercise, squeeze your legs together and pull your navel to your spine.

4. After six rockings, catch yourself with your palms.

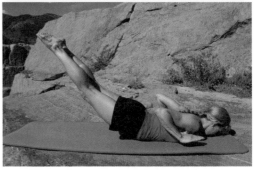

5. Counterpose this exercise by sitting back on your heels in Child's Pose (see page 212) to stretch your back.

Modifications: To modify this exercise, come up a shorter distance and make a smaller rocking motion. You may also consider substituting Swan Rocking for the exercise Skydiver.

Mat Maximizers

191

YOUR TOOLBOX

PURPOSE	DIFFICULTY	REPS
Strengthens the back and muscles along the spine. Stretches the chest and shoulders.	Beginner	5

1. This exercise is adapted from the Pilates reformer, where it is known as Pulling Straps from a T. Begin by lying on your stomach with your legs drawn together tightly and the inside edges of your feet touching. Bring your arms out to your sides like airplane wings, palms facing down. Place your forehead on the mat directly in front of you.

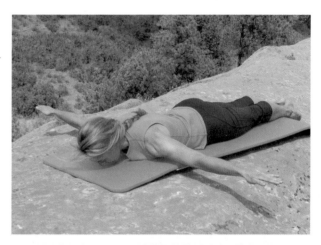

2. EXHALE all the air out of your lungs and pull your navel to your spine.

3. INHALE. Beginning from the top of your spine, lift your head and extend up through your spine. Simultaneously roll your shoulders back and draw your arms to your hips. Keep the tops of your feet anchored to the mat.

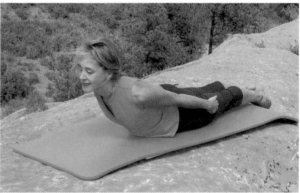

4. EXHALE; roll down and bring your arms back to start.

Extra Challenge: Use two- to three-pound dumbbells.

CORE Tree

PURPOSE	DIFFICULTY	REPS
Strengthens the abdominal muscles. Stretches iliotibial band, hamstrings, and hip extensors.	Intermediate 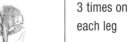	3 times on each leg

1. Lie on your back. Extend one leg along the mat and flex your foot. Extend the other leg straight up toward the sky with your foot pointed.

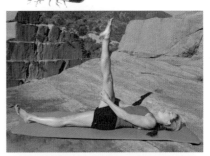

2. INHALE; lift your head and begin walking your hands up your leg, peeling your spine off the mat. Press through the heel of the foot on the floor to help keep the lower leg firmly anchored. EXHALE to come all the way up onto your sitz bones. Avoid pulling your shoulders up around your ears like a turtle.

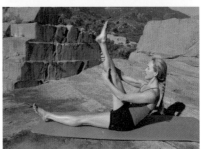

3. Take a full breath to roll back down. Keep your lower leg anchored to the mat like a tree root. Repeat 3 times.

4. At the top of the third time rolling up, place the opposite hand on the outside of your outer ankle, center yourself over

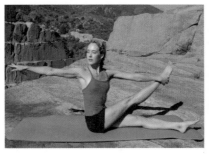 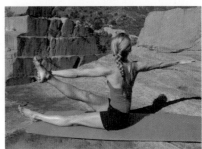

your sitz bones, lengthen your spine, and gently twist, opening up your chest to the side. Pretend someone is pulling you up by a string attached to your head. Lengthen out both sides of your waistline.

PURPOSE	DIFFICULTY	REPS
Strengthens the shoulders and arms.	Intermediate	10 forward, 10 reverse
Stretches the chest and shoulders.		
Challenges and improves balance.		

1. Begin by standing with your feet together and your arms by your sides.

2. With your palms facing up, INHALE and raise your arms up over your head and come up on the balls of your feet.

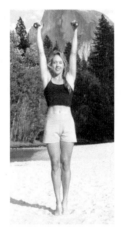
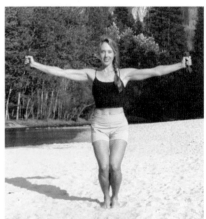

3. EXHALE and simultaneously bring your arms down to your sides, your heels down, and bend your knees. Pretend you are sliding your spine up and down against a wall as you lift up to your toes and come down and bend the knees. As your arms come down, keep your fingers within your peripheral vision. Keep your pelvis level and pull your navel to your spine.

4. Reverse the movement.

Modifications: For more stability, bring your feet hip-width apart.

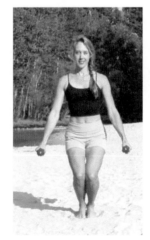
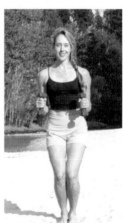

UPPER BODY Bug DUMBBELLS

PURPOSE	DIFFICULTY	REPS
Strengthens the back, shoulders, and arms.	Intermediate	10

1. Begin by standing with your feet together. Engage your core by pulling your navel to your spine. Bend your knees until you feel your hamstrings and hip flexors engage. Hinge at the hips until your back is parallel to the floor in a tabletop position. Make certain that your lower back doesn't arch. Make a circle with your arms in front of your chest so your palms face your chest and your knuckles touch. Draw your shoulders down and back. You should be looking straight down below your nose.

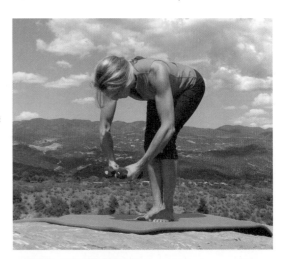

2. INHALE and raise your dumbbells out to the sides as if to open the circle. Draw your shoulder blades together. Your legs and torso stay completely still with your stomach drawn firm.

3. EXHALE; bring your arms back down into the circle in front of your chest.

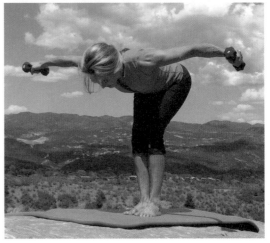

PURPOSE	DIFFICULTY	REPS
Strengthens the arms, shoulders, and abdominal muscles. Stretches hamstrings, shoulders, and back.	Intermediate	5

1. Begin by sitting with your legs out straight. Pretend you are sitting against a wall. Narrow your waistline and lift yourself tall, increasing the distance between your hips and ribs. Imagine there is a string attached to the crown of your head pulling you up. Bring your arms up to shoulder height and bend your elbows so that your palms face your forehead. Lift your sternum. Okay— you're ready to begin.

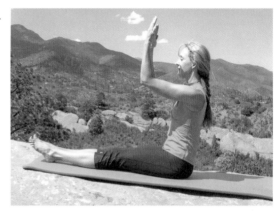

2. Pretend you are a bronze statue from the waist up. Draw your waistline tight. INHALE and hinge at your hips, only as far as you can while still keeping your heels on the mat.

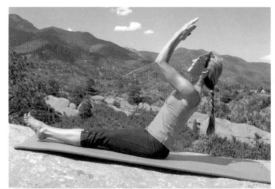

3. EXHALE; reach your arms straight forward and bend forward, head to knee.

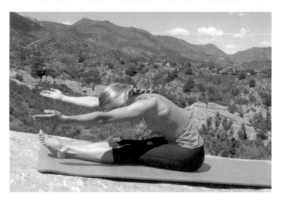

4. INHALE; row your arms out away from you as if you were pressing through water. Bring your arms behind your back, clasp your hands together, and roll your shoulders back so your shoulder blades slide down and back. If you're using dumbbells, you can omit the handclasp and bring your hands back to where the dumbbells just touch. Keep lifting your navel to your spine.

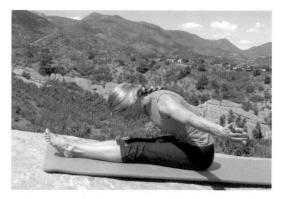

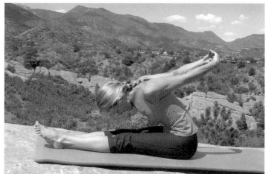

5. EXHALE; release your hands, rotate your arms from your shoulders so your palms face down, and stretch out over your legs. Pull your navel to your spine and from your tailbone, then curl back up, stacking your spine against the imaginary wall.

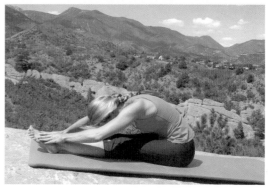

Modifications: If tight hamstrings make it difficult for you to sit up straight, roll up your mat and sit on it or sit on something (such as stacked books) to get you higher off the floor so your spine will be straight.

Extra Challenge: Use two- to three-pound dumbbells.

PURPOSE	DIFFICULTY	REPS
Strengthens the shoulders, chest, and back. Stretches the hamstrings and back. Improves posture.	Intermediate	5

1. Begin by sitting with your legs out straight. Pretend you are sitting against a wall. Narrow your waistline and lift yourself tall, stretching the distance between your ribs and hips. Imagine there is a string attached to the crown of your head pulling you up. Bring your arms to your sides so that your palms face the floor. Bring your thumbs by your ribs and pull your elbows back as if to touch them behind your back, drawing your shoulder blades down. Lift your sternum. Okay—you're ready to begin.

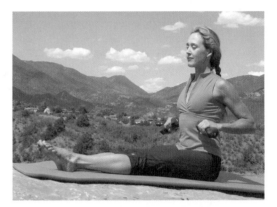

2. INHALE; reach your arms out straight to eye level. Keep your chest open, your collarbones reaching outward, and your lats engaged.

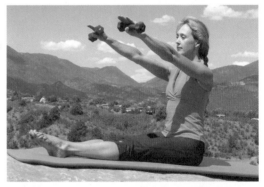

3. EXHALE; lower your arms straight to touch the mat. Continue to reach up tall through the crown of your head.

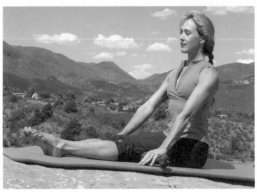

4. INHALE; raise your arms up toward the sky and keep your ribs knitted together.

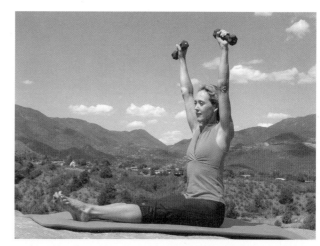

5. EXHALE; circle your arms out to the sides (making sure you can see your fingers in your peripherial vision) and back to start.

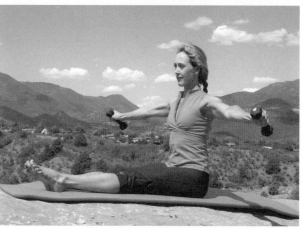

Modifications: If tight hamstrings make it difficult for you to sit up straight, roll up your mat and sit on it or sit on something (such as stacked books) to get you higher off the floor so your spine will be straight.

PURPOSE	DIFFICULTY	REPS
Strengthens the chest, shoulders, and arms.	Beginner	10

1. Begin with your legs crossed Indian style and your heels close to your sitz bones. Weight your sitz bones evenly. Pretend you are sitting against a wall. Narrow your waistline and lift yourself tall out of your hips. Imagine there is a string attached to the crown of your head pulling you up. Bring your arms out from your sides with your palms facing out. Pretend your arms are resting on an imaginary countertop. You should see your fingers in your peripheral vision.

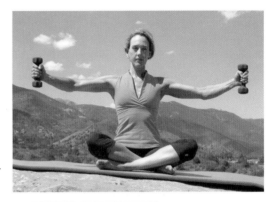

2. INHALE to prepare, EXHALE to bring the arms toward your centerline as if you were hugging a friend.

3. INHALE to open the circle, EXHALE to hug.

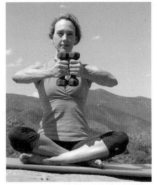

Modifications: If tight hips make it difficult for you to sit up straight, come to your knees or roll up your mat and sit on it or sit on something (such as stacked books) to get you higher off the floor so your spine will be straight.

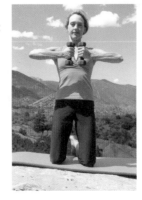
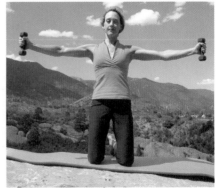

UPPER BODY Rotator Cuff DUMBBELLS

PURPOSE	DIFFICULTY	REPS
Strengthens the rotator cuff muscles. A must for climbers and paddlers.	Beginner	20 on each side

1. Lying on your side, stack your hips and shoulders and bend your knees in at a right angle. Bend your top arm at a 45-degree angle with your elbow on your hip.

2. INHALE and externally rotate your arm from your elbow so your hand moves away from your body.

3. EXHALE and release it down slowly with control to the starting position.

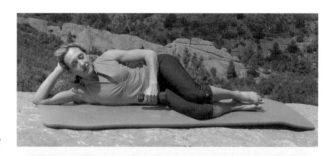

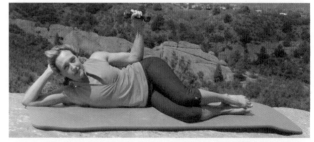

4. Maintain your sideline position, place the dumbbell in the hand of your lower arm. INHALE and internally rotate your arm from the elbow so that your palm comes up toward your shoulder. EXHALE and release it down slowly with control.

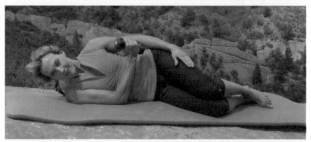

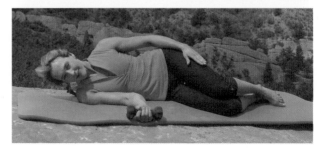

UPPER BODY Round Back DUMBBELLS OPTIONAL

PURPOSE	DIFFICULTY	REPS
Strengthens the arms, shoulders, and abdominal muscles.	Intermediate	5

1. Begin by sitting with your legs out straight. Pretend you are sitting against a wall. Narrow your waistline and lift yourself tall out of your hips. Imagine there is a string attached to the crown of your head pulling you up. Bring your arms in front of you, making a circle shape with your palms facing in. Lift your sternum. Okay—you're ready to begin.

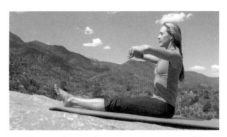

2. INHALE and tip your hips, curling your lower spine forward and rolling halfway down to the mat to the point before your heels lift.

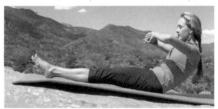

3. EXHALE and press your arms out to the side and curl your nose to your navel and head to knee.

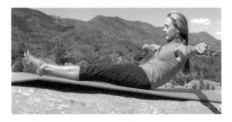

4. INHALE and bring your arms behind your back, clasp your hands together, and roll your shoulders back so that your shoulder blades are drawn close together. If you're using dumbbells, you can omit the handclasp and bring your hands back to where the dumbbells just touch. Keep lifting your navel to your spine.

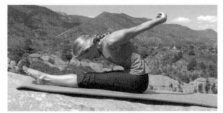

5. EXHALE; release your hands, rotate your arms from your shoulders so that your palms face down and stretch out over your legs. From your tailbone, curl back up, stacking your spine against the imaginary wall.

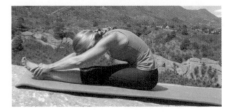

Modifications: If tight hamstrings make it difficult for you to sit up straight, roll up your mat and sit on it or sit on something (such as stacked books) to get you higher off the floor so your spine will be straight.

UPPER BODY Shaving the Head DUMBBELLS

PURPOSE	DIFFICULTY	REPS
Strengthens the triceps.	Intermediate	10
Stretches the hip extensors.		

1. Begin by sitting with your legs crossed and your heels close to your sitz bones. Try sitting with your legs crossed the opposite way you normally would. Weight your sitz bones equally and pretend you are sitting against a wall. Pull your abdominals in and upward creating a scooped-out waist and lift yourself tall out of your hips. Imagine there is a string attached to the crown of your head pulling you up. Bend your arms and bring your hands behind the nape of your neck. From your hips, hinge your spine forward so you feel a stretch in your hips. Avoid rounding your back or sinking into your chest. Keep your head in line with your spine.

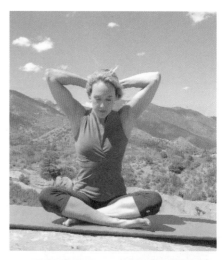

2. INHALE and straighten your arms up.

3. EXHALE and bend your elbows out wide and bring your hands back down to the nape of your neck.

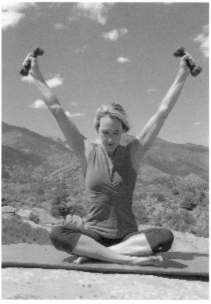

Side Bend Arms

PURPOSE	DIFFICULTY	REPS
Strengthens the shoulders and triceps. Stretches the obliques and hip flexors.	Intermediate	10 on each side

1. Begin by kneeling with your knees hip-width apart and your feet in a "V," heels together. Stack your knees, hips, and shoulders. Draw your shoulders down and back, pull your navel to your spine, and engage your hamstrings and outer hip muscles. Pretend your hips are pressed against an imaginary half wall. Bend sideways until your hand is on the ground. If needed, place a block or book beneath your hand. It is more important to keep a clean side bend than to create a deep bend.

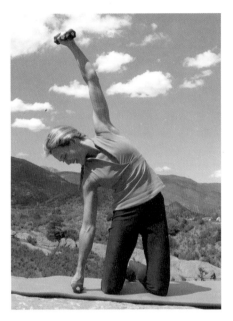

2. Bring the opposite arm over your head with your elbow bent and your palm facing the floor. INHALE and extend your arm to the sky. Keep your elbow stationary.

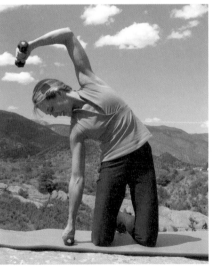

UPPER BODY Side-to-Side DUMBBELLS

PURPOSE	DIFFICULTY	REPS
Strengthens the abdominal muscles and shoulders.	Beginner	3–5 to each side
Stretches the waistline, back muscles, and shoulders.		

1. Begin by standing with your legs together and your arms by your sides. Energize your legs by squeezing them together and drawing your kneecaps upward. Bring one arm up by your ear and keep the other arm down by your side. Keep your pelvis level and pull your navel to your spine. Center your weight evenly between both feet and strive to keep it that way throughout the exercise. Take a deep INHALE and stretch up tall out of your hips, then bend your body sideways like a crescent moon, toward the arm at your side.

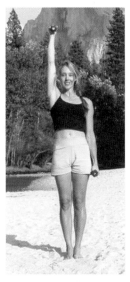

2. EXHALE, stretch the raised arm over your head, and allow your hips to reach out to opposite sides. Use oppositional energy to get maximum effectiveness out of this exercise. As you deepen the crescent moon shape, keep your hips and shoulders squared as if you were trapped between a screen and patio door. You should feel both stretching and strengthening of your waistline muscles and stretching of your hip flexors. Avoid shortening either side of your waist by continuously lifting out of your hips.

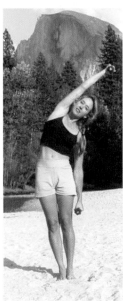
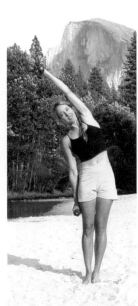

UPPER BODY Slide and Dive DUMBBELLS OPTIONAL

PURPOSE	DIFFICULTY	REPS
Strengthen the shoulders, arms, and back.	Intermediate	5
Stretches the hamstrings and back.		
Improves posture and articulates the spine.		

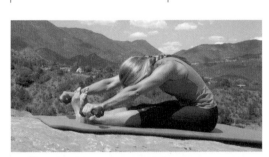

1. Begin by sitting with your legs out straight. Pretend you are sitting against a wall. Narrow your waistline and lift yourself tall out of your hips. Imagine there is a string attached to the crown of your head pulling you up. Bring your arms down by your sides with your elbows pointed directly back. Lift your sternum. Okay—you're ready to begin.

2. INHALE; curl your nose to your navel, like a snail curling into its shell, and hollow out your stomach. Slide your hands forward along the mat.

3. EXHALE; stack your spine tall against the imaginary wall, and allow your arms to float up like sleepwalker arms until your hands are shoulder height.

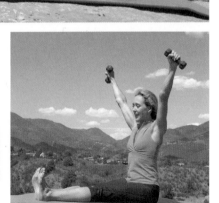

4. INHALE; raise your arms up toward the sky. EXHALE; circle your arms out to the sides (keep your hands in your peripheral vision), and back to start.

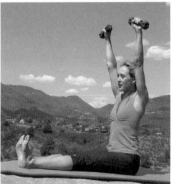
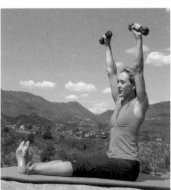

Modifications: If tight hamstrings make it difficult for you to sit up straight, sit on something to get you higher off the floor so your spine will be straight.

UPPER BODY Star

PURPOSE	DIFFICULTY	REPS
Strengthens the shoulders, arms, and abdominal muscles. Improves balance.	Advanced	1 on each side

1. This exercise has been adapted from the Pilates reformer. Sitting on one hip, extend your legs out straight with your top foot on the floor in front of your bottom foot. Your bottom arm is supporting you, palm flat on the floor.

2. INHALE and press up. Make yourself straight as an arrow in a side plank. Your supporting arm should be directly under your shoulder.

3. EXHALE and extend your top leg and arm up. Maintain your side plank and avoid sinking into your shoulders. Pretend you are between two panes of glass.

4. INHALE, bringing your top arm and leg back down.

5. EXHALE and lower yourself down to just a few inches off the floor. Avoid sitting down before you press back up. Avoid sinking into your shoulders.

Extra Challenge: From your side plank, sweep your top leg and arm forward, then back to center. Then scissor your top leg back and your top arm forward, then back to center.

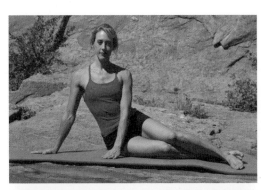

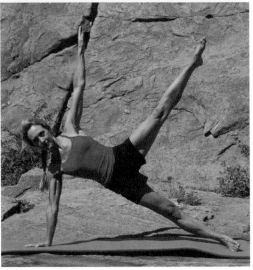

Triceps Kickbacks

PURPOSE	DIFFICULTY	REPS
Strengthens the arms (triceps).	Beginner	10
Strengthens hamstrings and hip extensors.		
Balances out the upper-arm muscles.		

1. Begin by standing with your feet together. Engage your core by pulling your navel to your spine. Bend your knees until you feel your hamstrings and hip flexors engage. Bring your back down until it's parallel to the floor in a tabletop position. Make certain that your lower back doesn't arch. You should be looking straight down below your nose. Bend your arms and bring your elbows in by your sides and your hands under your shoulders. Draw your shoulders down and back.

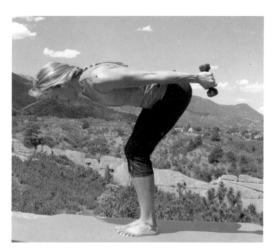

2. INHALE and straighten your arms, pressing the dumbbells up by your hips. Your legs and torso stay completely still with your stomach drawn firm.

3. EXHALE, bend your arms, and bring your hands back under your shoulders.

Modifications: An alternative to this exercise is Shaving the Head for the arms and Side Lunges for the legs.

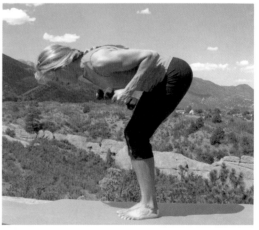

UPPER BODY Wrist Curls DUMBBELLS

PURPOSE	DIFFICULTY	REPS
Strengthens the forearm flexors and extensors.	Beginner	10–20 on each side

1. This exercise can be done kneeling, seated, or standing. It is important that you rest the inside of your forearm on a stable surface to create a neutral position for your wrist. This will help you monitor the extension and flexion of your wrist.

2. INHALE and curl your wrist, bringing the back of your hand closer to the back of your forearm.

3. EXHALE to slowly release with control. Repeat 20 times.

4. Turn your arm over.

5. INHALE and curl your wrist, bringing the palm of your hand closer to the front of your forearm.

6. EXHALE to slowly release with control. Repeat 20 times.

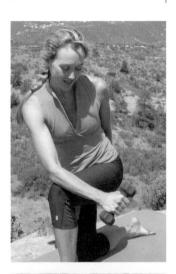

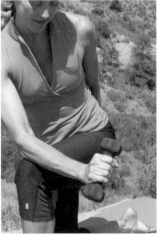

PURPOSE	DIFFICULTY	REPS
Strengthens the shoulders and arms.	Beginner	10

1. Begin by standing with your legs together and your arms by your sides. Energize your legs by squeezing them together and drawing your kneecaps upward. Center your arms in front of your legs with your palms facing your body.

2. INHALE and raise the dumbbells up, directing your elbows out to the sides. The dumbbells should remain in contact with each other as you bring them up below your chin.

3. EXHALE and lower the dumbbells down to the starting position. Make certain that you maintain proper alignment from your feet all the way to the top of your head while you do this exercise. For more challenge, bend your knees as you lower the dumbbells and come up to the balls of your feet as you raise them.

Modifications: To modify this exercise, use lighter dumbbells or omit the exercise altogether.

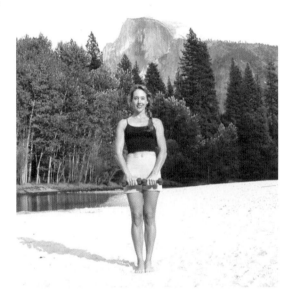

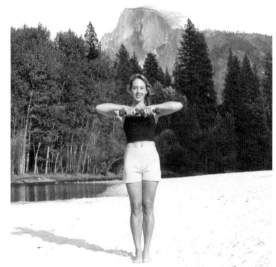

Chapter 15

Stretch Yourself

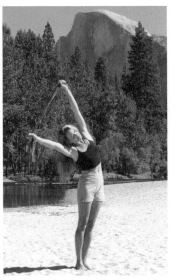

This chapter includes 19 Pilates-based stretches that are great warm-ups and cooldowns for all of your outdoor sports. Some stretches may require a stretch band. A jump rope, four-foot long cord, or bath towel can be used as well.

The following stretches are most effective when held for approximately 30 seconds to a minute. A good way to time your stretches is by the number of deep breaths you take on average in 30 seconds to a minute. This varies from person to person. Maintain an even breath on the inhale and the exhale.

Calves Stretch

PURPOSE

Stretches the Achilles tendon and calves (gastronemius and soleus muscles).

This stretch is extra important for runners, hikers, cyclists, and climbers.

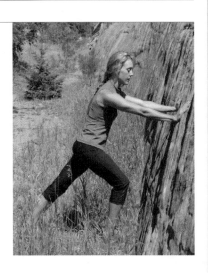

1. Stand an arm's distance from a wall and square your hips.

2. Place your hands on the wall in front of you and take a big step back with one leg while bending the front leg.

3. Press your back heel down. Engage your core and avoid arching your lower back.

4. Switch legs.

Child's Pose

PURPOSE

Stretches back, hip extensors, and shoulders.

1. Begin on your hands and knees, with knees hip-width apart.

2. Sit back on your heels, arms outstretched over your head. Allow your spine and the back of your shoulders to lengthen. If this is uncomfortable for your shoulders, bring your arms down by your sides.

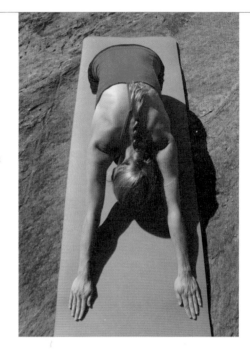

Figure 4

PURPOSE

Stretches your hip extensors and back.

1. Begin by lying on your back with your knees bent.

2. Cross your left ankle over your right knee.

3. Reach behind the right thigh and pull your leg toward your chest.

4. Keep the nape of your neck lengthened by gently nodding your chin toward your chest.

5. Repeat on other side.

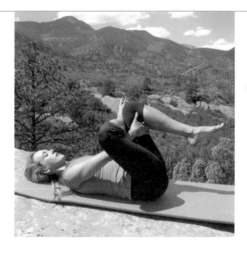

Figure 4 WITH SKI POLES OR HIKING POLES

PURPOSE

Stretches the hip extensors and back.

1. Place the poles in front of you for support and balance, holding them with both hands.

2. Cross one ankle over the opposite knee.

3. Keep your spine straight and gently bend your knees as if sliding your back down a wall.

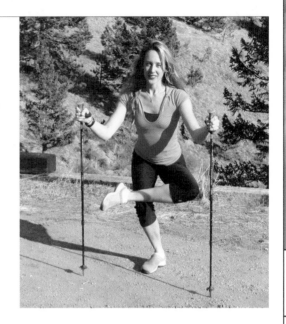

Forearm Stretch

PURPOSE

Stretches the forearm and hand extensors and flexors.

1. Straighten one arm, palm down, and gently pull your fingers toward the back of your arm until you feel your forearm stretch.

2. Release the stretch.

3. Flip your arm over so the palm is facing up and gently pull your fingers toward the bottom side of your forearm until you feel a stretch.

4. Switch arms.

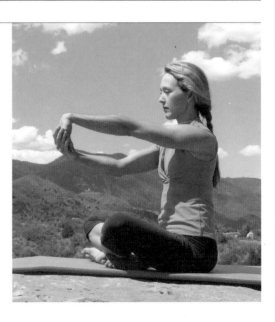

Leg Stretch WITH BAND

PURPOSE

Stretches the iliotibial bands, inner thighs, hamstrings, and hip flexors and extensors.

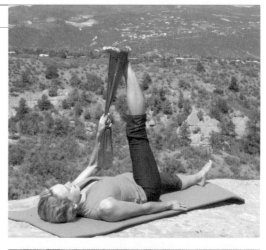

1. Begin by lying on your back with your legs out straight. Bring one leg toward your chest and place the stretch band beneath the sole of your foot. Gently lengthen the leg upward, pressing through the heel. Keep your shoulders down and the back of your neck lengthened.

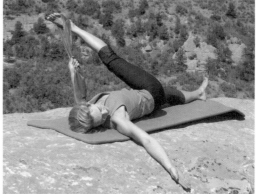

2. From the first position, gently pull your leg across the midline of your body until you feel a stretch along the outside of your leg and into the back of your hip. Hold the stretch band with the opposite hand.

3. Come back to center with your leg. Switch hands so you are holding the stretch band on the same side as the leg you are stretching. Open the leg to the side until you feel an inner thigh stretch.

4. Switch legs.

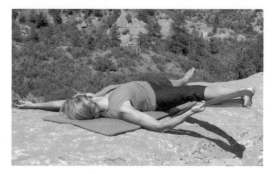

Mermaid

PURPOSE

Stretches the obliques, shoulders, and hips.

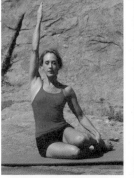
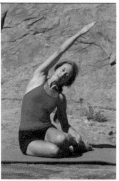

1. Sitting on your mat, bend your knees to the side. Stack your knees and ankles.

2. Hold on to your top ankle with the hand closest. Bring the other arm up by your ear.

3. INHALE; stretch your raised arm up over your head in the direction of your feet.

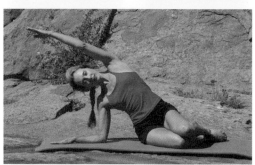

4. EXHALE up to center and bring the top hand down to the floor and the hand that held the ankle up toward the sky.

5. INHALE and side bend away from your feet.

6. Repeat 3 times in each direction.

Extra Challenge: To increase the hip stretch, cross your leg and place your top foot beside your knee.

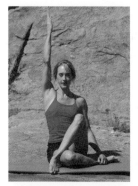
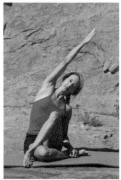

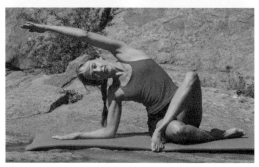

Neck Roll

PURPOSE

Stretches the neck, chest, abdominal muscles, and hip flexors.

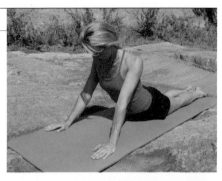

1. Begin by lying on your stomach with your hands under your shoulders. Draw your legs tightly together. Pull your tailbone toward your belly button. Engage your core.

2. INHALE. Beginning from the top your head, curl your spine up. Gently press up through the palms of your hands.

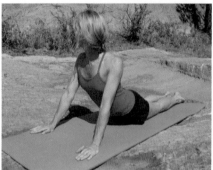

3. EXHALE to complete. Lift your sternum and draw your shoulders down and back. Your chin should be level and your forehead perpendicular with the floor.

4. Turn your head to the right.

5. Turn your head left, imagining that you are drawing a half circle with your nose.

Pigeon Pose

PURPOSE

Stretches your hip extensors.

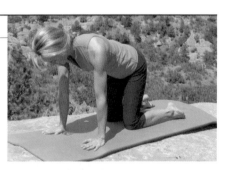

1. Begin on your hands and knees with your shoulders slightly behind your hands.

2. Bring your right knee toward your right wrist and angle your ankle toward your left wrist.

3. Slide your left leg behind you back so the front of your thigh is on the floor.

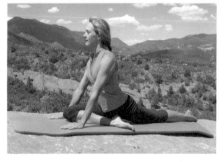

4. Press up with your arms, draw your shoulders down, and lift your sternum. You may also do this stretch by lowering your torso and resting it on your inner thigh. Keep your core engaged.

5. Switch sides.

Quadriceps Stretch

PURPOSE

Stretches your quadriceps, hip flexors, abdominal muscles, front of the shoulders, and chest.

1. Lying on your stomach, bend one leg, reach around with the opposite hand, and grab your ankle. Engage your core by pulling your navel to your spine.

2. Hold for 15 seconds.

3. Switch sides.

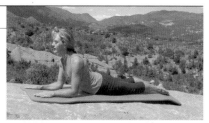
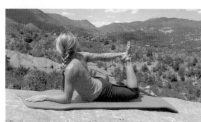
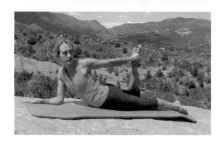

Rhomboid Stretch

PURPOSE

Stretches the muscles between your shoulder blades.

1. Bring one arm straight out front at shoulder height and bend your elbow at a 90-degree angle.

2. Bring the other arm up and wrap it around the first arm until your palms touch.

3. Press your palms together.

4. Lift your sternum and gently pull your elbows down.

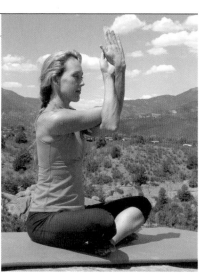

Shoulder Stretch

PURPOSE

Stretches the back of the shoulder.

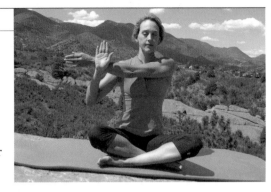

1. Bring one arm out straight in front of you.

2. Place the opposite hand on the outside of your arm and gently pull the arm across your body.

3. Switch.

Two-Minute Tailgate Stretches

PURPOSE

Stretches the hamstrings, quadriceps, hip extensors and flexors.

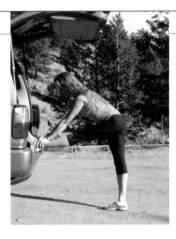

1. These stretches can easily be done off tailgates, bumpers, picnic tables, benches, and more. Begin by facing the tailgate. Raise one leg, place your heel on the top of the tailgate, leg out straight, and square your hips. The knee of your raised leg should point upward. The toes of your standing leg should point forward. INHALE and clasp your hands over your head. EXHALE and curl forward over your leg. Grab your foot if possible. Come back up.

2. Rotate on your standing leg until you are facing sideways and your raised leg is externally rotated. The kneecap should still face upward. INHALE and bring your outside arm up by your head. EXHALE and side bend toward your raised leg. Pretend that your back is against a wall and slide against it as you side bend. Keep your chest lifted and breathe.

3. Switch legs.

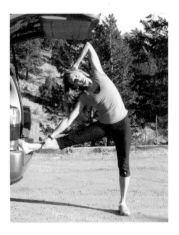

Triceps Stretch

PURPOSE

Stretches the triceps.

1. Lift one arm straight up over your head.

2. Bend your elbow so your palm falls back behind your head in between your shoulder blades. With the opposite hand, gently pull the elbow across.

3. Switch arms.

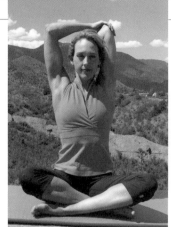
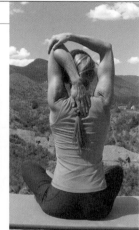

Upper-Body Band Stretches

PURPOSE

Stretches the shoulders, chest, and abdominals.

1. Stand with your feet together and bring the stretch band over your head.

2. Lift your sternum and gently bend sideways into a crescent moon shape. Keep your hips and shoulders square as if you were between two panes of glass.

3. Repeat on the opposite side.

4. Come back to center. Lift your sternum and bring the band behind your head.

Note: It is possible to do these stretches seated as well.

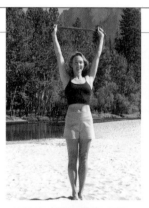
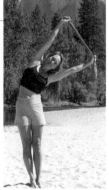
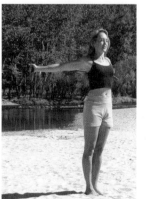

Wall Stretch

PURPOSE

Stretches hamstrings and hip extensors.

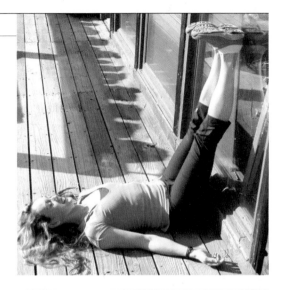

1. Lie down on your back and place your legs up against a wall.

2. Scoot your body close to the wall, placing your sitz bones as close to the wall as possible while still keeping your tailbone on the floor.

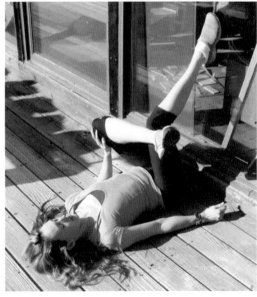

3. Cross your ankle to your opposite knee and avoid shifting your hips or shortening your waist.

4. Switch legs.

Partner Stretches

The following stretches are designed to be done with a partner. Whenever you are stretching someone, make certain that he or she has the best possible spine and joint alignment. Likewise, if someone is stretching you, honor your alignment before going for a deeper stretch.

Partner Child's Pose

PURPOSE

Stretches the back and hip extensors.

1. As your partner performs Child's Pose, described on page 212, stand behind him and press gently on his hips. Avoid pressing on the lower back.

2. Ask for feedback to determine the appropriate level of pressure.

Partner Saw

PURPOSE

Stretches the hamstrings, torso, and shoulders.

1. To stretch your partner, stand behind her as she performs the Saw exercise as described on page 145 in Chapter 13.

2. As she saws her pinky finger past her pinky toe, gently place your foot on her opposite hip crease to hold the hip down and stretch the hamstring.

3. At the same time, press on the shoulder on the same side and gently pull back her arm. Again, do this gently and ask for feedback to determine the appropriate level of pressure.

Partner Tree

PURPOSE

To stretch the iliotibial band, hip extensors, and torso.

1. After your partner has created the final position of Tree (described on page 193), stand behind her and gently place your leg against her spine to provide support for better alignment.

2. As you do so, make sure that you are helping her sit taller and more evenly over both sitz bones. It may be necessary for your partner to bend the leg that she is holding in order to create this alignment.

3. Help her lift her chest by gently pulling her arms and shoulders back. Again, do this gently and ask for feedback to determine the appropriate level of pressure.

Stretch Yourself

221

YOUR TOOLBOX

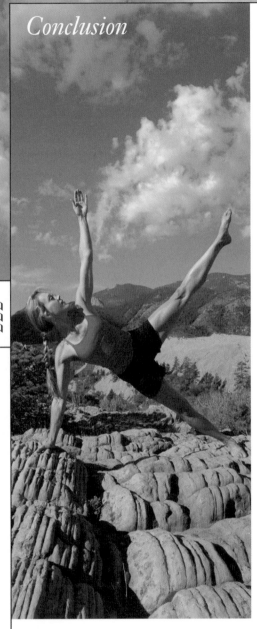

Conclusion

No matter if you are a cyclist, skier, or rock climber, performing your best, staying injury free, and maintaining longevity as an athlete are common goals among all of us. Regular Pilates practice will help you to achieve these goals without dependence on an athletic trainer or a gym. It is perfect if you are reasonably fit and want to the freedom to do the work on your own time and in your own space.

Whether you are discovering Pilates for the first time or taking your study to the next level, I hope that you have found the tools in this book valuable in your quest to stay active, fit, and injury free. As a mentor of mine used to say, "Sift all the information you have received through the colander of your mind and keep that which remains." As a fellow outdoor athlete, I wish you much health, happiness, and many more sunny days pursuing your passions under the great blue sky.

—Lauri

Appendix A

Pilates Exercise Reference Chart

EXERCISE	DIFFICULTY	STRENGTHENING	STRETCHING	PAGE
Arm Circles	Intermediate	Arms, Shoulders	Chest, Shoulders	194
Bicycle	Advanced	Abdominals, Shoulders, Arms	Hamstrings, Quadriceps, Hip Flexors	151
Boomerang	Intermediate	Abdominals	Back, Hamstrings, Shoulders	164
Bug	Intermediate	Back, Shoulders, Arms	N/A	195
Calves Stretch	Beginner	N/A	Achilles Tendon, Calves	211
Cancan	Intermediate	Abdominals, Hip Flexors	Hip Extensors	180
Captain Crunch	Intermediate	Abdominals	Hamstrings	181
Child's Pose	Beginner	N/A	Back, Hip Extensors, Shoulders	212
Control Balance	Advanced	Abdominals	Hamstrings	167
Coordination	Intermediate	Abdominals, Triceps	N/A	182
Corkscrew	Intermediate	Abdominals	Hip Extensors	144
Crisscross	Intermediate	Abdominals	Torso, Shoulders	183
Crossover	Advanced	Abdominals	Hamstrings	184

EXERCISE	DIFFICULTY	STRENGTHENING	STRETCHING	PAGE
Double-Leg Kick	Intermediate	Hamstrings, Hip Extensors, Back	Chest, Shoulders, Hip Flexors	148
Double-Leg Stretch	Beginner	Abdominals	Shoulders	140
Double-Straight-Leg Stretch	Intermediate	Abdominals	N/A	185
Elementary Backstroke	Intermediate	Abdominals, Arms	N/A	186
Figure 4	Beginner	N/A	Hip Extensors, Back	212
Flatback	Intermediate	Arms, Shoulders, Abdominals	Hamstrings, Shoulders, Back	196
Figure 4 with Ski Poles or Hiking Poles	Beginner	N/A	Hip Extensors, Back	213
Footwork	Intermediate	Abdominals, Inner Thighs	N/A	187
Forearm Stretch	Beginner	N/A	Forearms, Hand Extensors, Hand Flexors	213
Hip Circles	Advanced	Abdominals, Hip Flexors	Chest, Front of Shoulders	158
Hug a Tree	Beginner	Chest, Shoulders, Arms	N/A	200
The Hundred	Beginner	Abdominals, Triceps	N/A	130
Jackknife	Advanced	Abdominals, Shoulders	Hamstrings, Back	154
Kneeling Side Kicks	Advanced	Legs, Hips, Abdominals	N/A	162
Leg Pull-Up	Advanced	Shoulders, Arms, Quadriceps, Hip Flexors	Hamstrings, Hip Extensors, Chest	161
Leg Pull-Front	Intermediate	Shoulders, Hamstrings, Abdominals	Calves	160
Leg Stretch with Band	Beginner	N/A	Iliotibial Bands, Inner Thighs, Hamstrings, Hip Flexors, Extensors	214
Mermaid	Beginner	N/A	Obliques, Shoulders, Hips	215

EXERCISE	DIFFICULTY	STRENGTHENING	STRETCHING	PAGE
Neck Pull	Intermediate	Abdominals	Hamstrings, Back	149
Neck Roll	Intermediate	N/A	Neck, Chest, Abdominals, Hip Flexors	216
One-Leg Circles	Beginner	Abdominals, Quadriceps, Hip Flexors	Hip Extensors, Hamstrings, Iliotibial Band	136
One-Leg Kick	Beginner	Hamstrings, Hip Extensors	Abdominals, Hip Flexors, Quadriceps	147
One-Leg Push-Ups	Intermediate	Shoulders, Chest, Arms, Abdominals	Hamstrings, Back	170
One-Leg Stretch	Beginner	Abdominals	Hip Flexors	139
One-Straight-Leg Stretch	Beginner	Abdominals	Hamstrings, Hip Flexors	188
Open-Leg Rocker	Intermediate	Abdominals	Hamstrings, Back	142
Partner Child's Pose	Beginner	N/A	Back, Hip Extensors	221
Partner Saw	Beginner	N/A	Hamstrings, Torso, Shoulders	221
Partner Tree	Intermediate	N/A	Iliotibial Band, Hip Extensors, Torso	221
Pigeon Pose	Beginner	N/A	Hip Extensors	216
Push-Ups	Intermediate	Shoulders, Chest, Arms, Abdominals	Hamstrings, Back	168
Quadriceps Stretch	Beginner	N/A	Quadriceps, Hip Flexors, Abdominals, Front of Shoulders, Chest	217
Rhomboid Stretch	Beginner	N/A	Back	217
Roll Over	Intermediate	Abdominals, Shoulders, Triceps	Back, Hamstrings	134
Roll Up	Intermediate	Abdominals	Hamstrings, Back, Shoulders	132
Rolling Like a Ball	Beginner	Abdominals	Back	138
Rotator Cuff	Beginner	Rotator Cuffs	N/A	201

Pilates Exercise Reference Chart

225

MORE TOOLS

EXERCISE	DIFFICULTY	STRENGTHENING	STRETCHING	PAGE
Round Back	Intermediate	Arms, Shoulders, Abdominals	Hamstrings, Shoulders, Back	202
Rowing	Intermediate	Shoulders, Chest, Back	Hamstrings, Back	198
Saw	Beginner	Abdominals	Hamstrings, Torso	145
Scissors	Advanced	Abdominals, Shoulders, Arms	Hamstrings, Quadriceps, Hip Flexors	150
Seal	Beginner	Abdominals	Back, Hips	166
Shaving the Head	Intermediate	Triceps	Hip Extensors	203
Shoulder Bridge with Kicks	Beginner	Hamstrings, Back	Quadriceps, Hip Flexors	152
Shoulder Stretch	Beginner	N/A	Shoulders	218
Side Bend	Advanced	Abdominals, Shoulders	Abdominals, Hips	163
Side Bend Arms	Intermediate	Shoulders, Triceps	Obliques, Hip Flexors	204
Side-to-Side	Beginner	Abdominals, Shoulders	Waistline, Back, Shoulders	205
Side Kicks	Beginner	Legs, Hips	Legs, Hips	155
Side Kicks—Bicycle	Intermediate	Legs, Hips	Hips	177
Side Kicks—Circles	Intermediate	Legs, Hips	Hips	174
Side Kicks— Heel Clicks	Intermediate	Legs, Hips	Hips	178
Side Kicks— Inner Thigh	Intermediate	Legs, Hips	Hips	175
Side Kicks— Kick-Ups	Intermediate	Legs, Hips	Hips	173
Side Kicks— Lower-Leg Lifts	Intermediate	Legs, Hips	Hips	175
Side Kicks— Paintbrush	Intermediate	Legs, Hips	Hips	172

EXERCISE	DIFFICULTY	STRENGTHENING	STRETCHING	PAGE
Side Kicks— Scissors	Intermediate	Legs, Hips	Hips	176
Side Lunges	Beginner	Legs, Hips	Hip Flexors	179
Slide and Dive	Intermediate	Shoulders, Arms, Back	Hamstrings, Back	206
Skydiver	Intermediate	Back	N/A	189
Snake	Advanced	Back	Chest, Front of Shoulders	190
Spine Stretch	Beginner	Abdominals	Hamstrings, Back	141
Spine Twist	Intermediate	Abdominals	N/A	153
Star	Advanced	Shoulders, Arms, Abdominals	N/A	207
Swan Dive	Advanced	Back, Shoulders	Abdominals, Hip Flexors	146
Swan Rocking	Intermediate	Back, Shoulders	Abdominals, Hip Flexors	191
Swimming	Intermediate	Back, Shoulders	Abdominals, Hip Flexors	159
T-Bird	Beginner	Back	Chest, Shoulders	192
Teaser Series	All Levels	Abdominals, Hip Flexors, Quadriceps	N/A	156
Tree	Intermediate	Abdominals	Iliotibial Band, Hamstrings, Hip Extensors	193
Triceps Kickbacks	Beginner	Triceps	Hamstrings, Hip Extensors	208
Triceps Stretch	Beginner	N/A	Triceps	219
Two-Minute Tailgate Stretches	Beginner	N/A	Hamstrings, Quadriceps, Hip Extensors, Flexors	218
Upper-Body Band Stretches	Beginner	N/A	Shoulders, Chest, Abdominals	219
Wall Stretch	Beginner	N/A	Hamstrings, Hip Extensors	220
Wrist Curls	Beginner	Forearm Flexors, Extensors	N/A	209
Zip-Ups	Beginner	Shoulders, Arms	N/A	210

Appendix B
Create Your Own Pilates Prescription

Major Outdoor Sport: _____

Goal: _____

_____

_____

Formula: _____

_____

_____

Creating Balance

Muscles to Stretch: _____

_____

_____

_____

_____

Muscles to Strengthen: _____

_____

_____

_____

_____

To create your Pilates cross-training routine, select from four core-strengthening exercises, four strengthening exercises, and four stretching exercises from Appendix A. Alternate these routines three to five days per week, or supplement them with one of the full-body conditioning routines in Appendix D.

Routine A	Routine B
1.	1.
2.	2.
3.	3.
4.	4.
5.	5.
6.	6.
7.	7.
8.	8.
9.	9.
10.	10.
11.	11.
12.	12.

After-Training Stretches:

Appendix C
Common Injuries to Outdoor Athletes

Achilles Tendonitis

The Achilles tendon is the largest tendon in the human body and also the most frequently injured tendon. The Achilles tendon attaches to the heel bone (calcaneus) and connects the leg muscles to the foot. Achilles tendonitis is often characterized by pain felt a few inches about the heel bone after working out or in the morning. It can be caused by training errors, excessive foot pronation, and tight calf muscles (gastronemius and soleus). Regular stretching of the calves, smart training practices, and wearing proper footwear are your best defense against this injury.

AC (Acromioclavicular) Joint Separations

This injury can happen by landing on your shoulder or on an outstretched arm while skiing, snowboarding, or falling off your bike. The AC joint ligaments connect your collarbones to the tips of your shoulder blades. The force of a fall can cause these ligaments to separate.

Ankle Sprains

According to the American Academy of Orthopaedic Surgeons, approximately 25,000 people experience ankle sprains each day. They are commonly caused by excessive motion in the ankle joint. Running or hiking on uneven terrain can cause the ankle to suddenly roll in, stretching or tearing the ligaments of the ankle followed by acute pain, inflammation, and bruising. To avoid chronic ankle sprains, maintain uniform muscle balance and flexibility in your legs and hips. In addition, practice smart training habits and wear supportive shoes. To strengthen your ankles, try exercises such as picking up towels with your toes and writing the alphabet in the air with your big toe.

Anterior Cruciate Ligament (ACL) Injury

The ACL is one of four ligaments that function to stabilize the knee. The ACL stabilizes the knee and prevents hyperextension of the knee joint. Injury to the ACL can be caused by overuse due to poor alignment of the kneecap and by twisting or falling onto the knee. Injury to the ACL is more common in women than men due to their wider hips, greater knee flexibility, and higher degree of foot pronation. Strengthening the abdominals and hips can improve the alignment of the knees, thereby reducing internal knee rotation and the chances of an ACL injury. Maintaining equal muscle balance in the legs is also important.

Biceps Femoris Tendonitis

This is inflammation to the tendons of the hamstrings connecting muscle to bone in and around the knee. It can be caused by overuse and insufficient core strength. Pain may be felt when you bend your knee while using resistance.

Carpal Tunnel Syndrome

This is inflammation to the medial nerve of the wrist, sometimes experienced by cyclists from pressure applied by holding on to the handlebars. It results in tingling, numbness, or pain in the fingers and thumb. If you are a cyclist, you can minimize your risk for this injury by adjusting your bike position to take pressure off your hands and wrists. Also, wearing padded gloves and padding the handlebars helps to minimize shock. Forearm and hand stretches before and after riding are also recommended.

Chondromalacia

This is inflammation to the cartilage on the back side of the kneecap. Sharp pain is experienced beneath and in front of the kneecap. As the cartilage breaks down, crunching sounds and pain at the back of the knee may occur. Over time the knee becomes arthritic and is unable to cushion the joint. Muscle imbalances in the quadriceps muscles contribute to this injury. If the outer quadriceps muscle (lateral medialis) becomes stronger than the inner quadriceps muscle (vastus medialis), the integrity of the knee is compromised. Excessive pronation of the foot, a high Q-angle, and trail running over sloping terrain challenge the alignment of the kneecap and can create microtrauma in the joint.

De Quervains Disease (DQD)

This is an overuse injury to the tendons of the thumb and is experienced by mountain bikers from excessive braking and shifting of gears. Pain is felt on the inside of the wrist when making wrist and thumb movements.

Fallen Metatarsal Arch

Experts are uncertain what causes the arch to fall; however, a sudden increase in an athlete's intensity, frequency, and volume is suspected. This condition is characterized by pain under the ball of the foot and a foot that appears puffier than normal. Using softer shoes with more cushioning can sometimes help prevent this injury.

Finger Pulley Strain or Rupture

Characterized by partial tears or complete ruptures of the flexor tendon annular pulleys. This is a common overuse injury in climbers. When it occurs, it may be accompanied by a popping sound. Pain and swelling are present. For an in-depth discussion of this injury, please refer to *Training for Climbing* by Eric J. Hörst.

Herniated/Ruptured/Slipped Disc

This injury may occur over time through normal wear and tear. Cracks that develop in one or more discs of the spine result in the escape of fluid. As a result, the disc is unable to provide cushion and absorb shock. Pain may be felt if pressure from the herniated disc is placed on the nerve roots or spinal cord. Pain may be localized in the back or radiate down the leg into the foot; however, many people experience no symptoms at all.

Iliotibial-Band (ITB) Syndrome

The ITB runs down the side of the leg and connects from the hip to the lower outer leg bone. ITB Syndrome occurs when tendon tightness creates friction over the knobby bone on the outside of the knee. This overuse injury can be caused by poor foot biomechanics, weak lateral hip muscles, and overtraining. Strengthening the outer hip muscles while stretching the iliotibial band, hamstrings, and calves go a long way toward preventing ITB Syndrome.

Lateral Epicondylitis (Tennis Elbow)

Pain on the outside bump of the elbow may be experienced while turning doorknobs or grabbing objects. Injury occurs when forearm flexor muscles become stronger than the extensors. Maintaining healthy elbows means proper cross-training exercise to create and maintain uniform muscle balance in the upper arm and forearm. Reverse wrist curls and triceps strengtheners are important cross-training exercises to avoid this injury.

Medial Collateral Ligament (MCL) Injury

The MCL is on the inner side of the knee and is one of four ligaments that function to stabilize the knee. It can be torn due to pressure placed on the inside of the knee, such as while snowplowing. It is not uncommon for this injury to be accompanied by injury to the ACL. Symptoms include pain, swelling, and bruising along the inside of the knee.

Medial Epicondylitis (Golfer's Elbow)

This overuse injury is often caused by muscle imbalances. It affects the flexor muscles and tendons of the forearms. Pain may be felt on the inside of the elbow when making a fist and squeezing. Pronator exercises and adequate rest between workouts are important cross-training to avoid this injury.

Meniscus Injuries

The meniscus is made up of cartilage and provides shock absorption and cushioning at the knee joint between the femur and the tibia.

Tenderness, swelling, and a feeling of the knee giving way are sometimes experienced. Like MCL and ACL injuries, meniscus injuries occur due to twisting motion and repetitive bending. Maintaining muscle balance in the legs is the best preventive cross-training for this injury. Strengthening the quadriceps and stretching the hamstrings is recommended.

Patella Tendonitis (Jumper's Knee)

This is inflammation to the front tendon that connects the kneecap to the shinbone. It is often caused by overuse, especially from jumping activities associated with sports such as running and skiing. Repetitive impact and overuse can lead to inflammation of the anterior (front) tendon connecting the kneecap to the shinbone. Pain may be felt just below the kneecap when pedaling a bicycle or walking upstairs or squatting, and the area may be tender to the touch. Pushing too big of a gear while cycling or taking on too many moguls while skiing can contribute to this condition. Maintaining uniform muscle balance in quadriceps and hamstrings, wearing proper footwear, and smart training practices are key to avoiding this injury.

Patellofemoral Pain Syndrome (Runner's Knee)

This overuse injury is common among runners, cyclists, skiers, and female athletes with high Q-angles. It is often caused by misalignment of the kneecap, injury, overuse, and muscle imbalance. As the cartilage of the kneecap begins to wear out, pain is felt under and around the kneecap. People with Patellofemoral Pain Syndrome may experience pain and stiffness while going up and down stairs, after sitting for a long time, and while squatting and kneeling. Maintaining uniform muscle balance between the quadriceps and hamstrings is key to preventing this injury.

Plantar Fasciitis

Caused by overly tight calves and an over-pronating foot, plantar fasciitis causes the fibrous tissue of the foot to be pulled and torn. "Plantar" refers to the bottom of your foot, "fascia" refers to the connective tissue, and "itis" refers to its condition: inflamed. Heel spurs develop, and pain is experienced under the heel or the arch of the foot, typically in the morning or after sitting for a long time. Muscle imbalances and overuse can lead to this injury. Exercises such as picking up towels with your toes, toe raises, and stretching your calves can help prevent this injury.

Plica Syndrome

This overuse injury creates inflammation to the synovial tissue lining inside the knee. It is marked by pain on the medial side of the knee and by stiffness and sharp pain when straightening the leg after sitting. Maintaining muscle balance in the leg is the best preventive cross-training for this injury. Strengthening the quadriceps and stretching the hamstrings are recommended.

Rotator Cuff Tendonitis (Swimmer's Shoulder)

Swimmer's shoulder is tendonitis to the rotator cuff muscles, often caused by swimming too much or bad technique. In doing so, muscle imbalances in the shoulders and back are created. Impingement occurs in the rotator cuff and creates inflammation leading to tendonitis.

Sciatica

Sciatica is caused by pressure on the sciatic nerve and is characterized by pain in the lower back that radiates through the buttocks, down the outside of the leg, and sometimes all the way to the toes. Factors such as running without proper core engagement, poor posture, and lifting heavy objects by bending at the back instead of at the knees are just a few of the ways athletes put excessive pressure on the lumbar disks of their spine. Structural misalignments, such as one leg being longer than the other, can wreak havoc on the sciatic nerve as well. Improving your posture, strengthening the muscles of your core, and improving your hamstring flexibility are strategies for avoiding sciatica.

Shermer's Neck

This injury was named after a cyclist named Michael Shermer in 1983. It is caused by muscle fatigue of the neck extensor muscles due to holding the head up while cycling in an aerodynamic position. It is more common in long-distance cyclists. The symptoms include pain in the back of the neck followed by difficulty holding the head up. Sufferers may resort to propping up the head with neck braces and chin devices.

Shin Splints

What begins as inflammation to the outer lining of the bone and soft tissues can progress into a stress fracture to the lower leg bones (tibia and fibula). Weekend warriors, those who run too hard, too fast, and violate the 10 percent per week progression rule, may fall victim to shin splints. Shin splints occur when your muscles develop faster than the bones can keep up. Running on hard surfaces and skiing the bumps develop overly tight calves and contribute to this injury.

Shoulder Impingement

Shoulder impingement occurs when the supraspinatus tendon that runs along the top of your shoulder gets pinched. It is characterized by inflammation that can lead to tendonitis. Symptoms include feeling a painful pinching sensation when the arm is raised over the head. It is often caused by overuse or muscle imbalances in the rotator cuff muscles.

Shoulder Subluxation

A partial dislocation that results from muscle imbalances and overstretched ligaments, subluxation shows up as deep pain in the back of the shoulder and sometimes requires surgery to tighten the loosened ligaments and tendons.

Talus Injuries

Fractures and sprains to the ankle, specifically the lateral process of the talus (LPT) are most common to snowboarders. The LPT is a wedge-shaped bone that assists in rotation and hinge movement of the ankle. Snowboarders who wear soft lace-up boots are more likely to injure their ankles than riders wearing hard boots.

Ulnar Collateral Ligament of the Thumb Injury (Skier's Thumb)

This injury occurs to skiers who fall with their hands improperly looped through their ski pole straps. During a fall, excessive force is placed on the ulnar collateral ligaments of the thumb, causing the thumb to bend excessively backward and outward, resulting in injury.

Ulnar Neuritis (Handlebar Palsy)

This injury is more common in cyclists, due to the pressure placed on the wrist, and in sports requiring the elbow to be bent for long periods of time. Compression is created on the ulnar nerve, creating pain and numbness on the inside of the elbow that radiates down into the fourth and fifth fingers. Sufferers usually experience loss of strength in the hands. To avoid ulnar neuritis, it is a good idea to have your cycling position evaluated by a professional and consider padding your handlebars and wearing biking gloves to provide cushioning and alleviate pressure. Using neutral wrist positions that minimize pressure and performing forearm stretches before and after rides are recommended.

Ulnar Nerve Entrapment

This injury to the inside of the elbow at the "funny bone" (the ulnar nerve) often results from elbow misalignment leading to stretching of the ulnar nerve. Pain and numbness in the forearm are accompanied by pain radiating down into the ring and pinky finger.

Whiplash

Also known as a neck sprain or strain, whiplash causes injury to the soft tissues of the neck. It is usually caused by sudden extension (backward movement of the neck) and flexion (forward movement of the neck). Snowboarders who fall on hard-packed ice sometimes experience neck injuries similar to those sustained when rear-ended in an automobile accident.

Appendix D

Additional Pilates Routines

General Conditioning

The following routines are designed to be general-conditioning routines that can be done in addition to or instead of the 15-minute sports-specific routines. These routines require 15 to 45 minutes and are not sport specific.

Level 1
Basic Routine

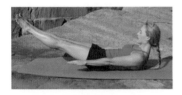

1. The Hundred, page 130

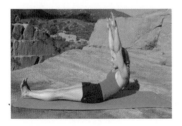

2. Roll Up, page 132

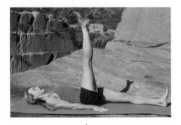

3. One-Leg Circles, page 136

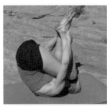

4. Rolling Like a Ball, page 138

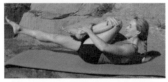

5. One-Leg Stretch, page 139

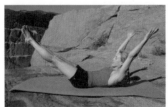

6. Double-Leg Stretch, page 140

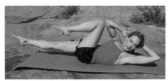

7. Crisscross, page 183

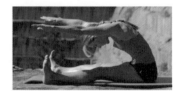

8. Spine Stretch, page 141

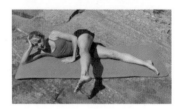

9. Side Kicks Series, pages 171–178

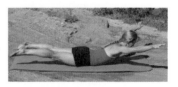

10. Skydiver, page 189

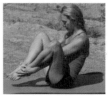

11. Seal, page 166

Level 2
Intermediate Routine

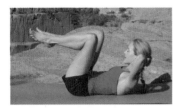

1. Footwork, page 187

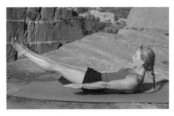

2. The Hundred, page 130

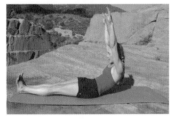

3. Roll Up, page 132

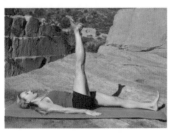

4. One-Leg Circles, page 136

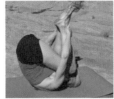

5. Rolling Like a Ball, page 138

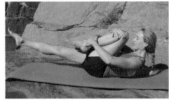

6. One-Leg Stretch, page 139

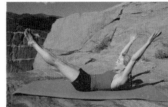

7. Double-Leg Stretch, page 140

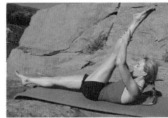

8. One-Straight-Leg Stretch, page 188

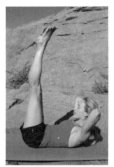

9. Double-Straight-Leg Stretch, page 185

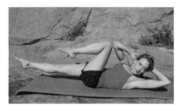

10. Crisscross, page 183

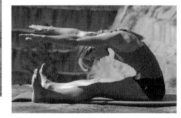

11. Spine Stretch, page 141

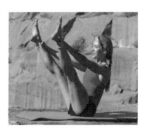

12. Open-Leg Rocker, page 142

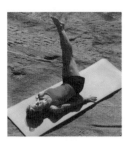

13. Corkscrew, page 144

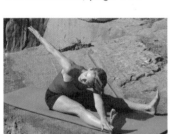

14. Saw, page 145

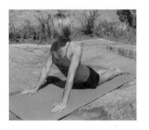

15. Neck Roll, page 216

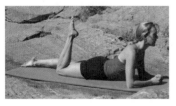

16. One-Leg Kick, page 147

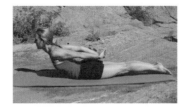

17. Double-Leg Kick, page 148

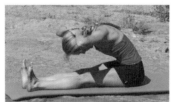

18. Neck Pull, page 149

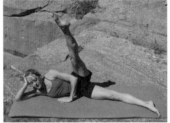

19. Side Kick Series, page 171–178

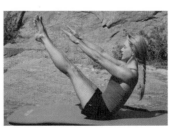

20. Teaser Series, page 156

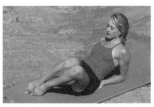

21. Cancan, page 180

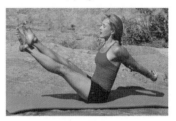

22. Boomerang, page 164

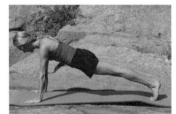

23. Push-Ups, page 168

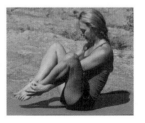

24. Seal, page 166

Level 3
Advanced Routine

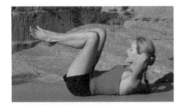

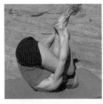

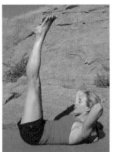

10.
Double-
Straight-
Leg
Stretch,
page
185

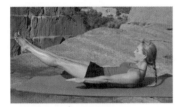

6.
Rolling
Like a Ball,
page 138

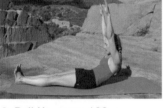

1. Footwork, page 187

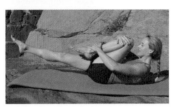

2. The Hundred, page 130

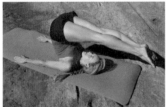

7. One-Leg Stretch, page 139

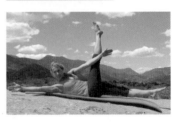

11. Crossover, page 184

3. Roll Up, page 132

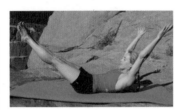

8. Double-Leg Stretch,
page 140

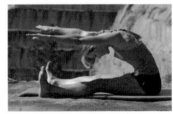

12. Spine Stretch, page 141

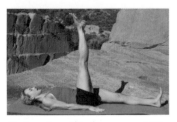

4. Roll Over, page 134

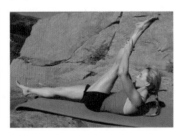

9. One-Straight-Leg Stretch,
page 188

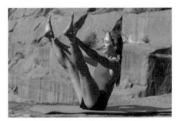

13. Open-Leg Rocker,
page 142

5. One-Leg Circles, page 136

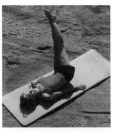

14. Cork-screw, page 144

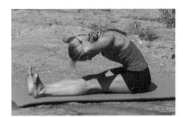

19. Neck Pull, page 149

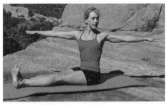

23. Spine Twist, page 153

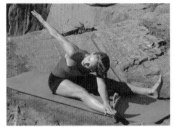

15. Saw, page 145

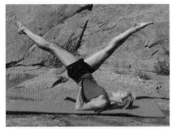

20. Scissors, page 150

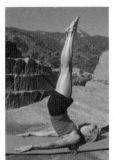

24. Jack-knife, page 154

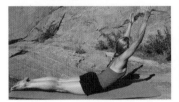

16. Swan Dive, page 146

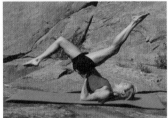

21. Bicycle, page 151

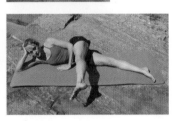

25. Side Kick Series, pages 171–178

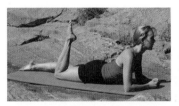

17. One-Leg Kick, page 147

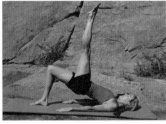

22. Shoulder Bridge with Kicks, page 152

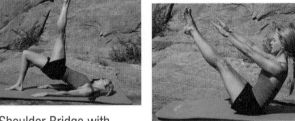

26. Teaser Series, page 156

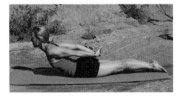

18. Double-Leg Kick, page 148

Additional Pilates Routines

239

MORE TOOLS

Level 3
Advanced Routine (continued)

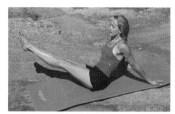

27. Hip Circles, page 158

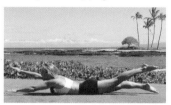

28. Swimming, page 159

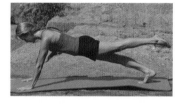

29. Leg Pull-Front, page 160

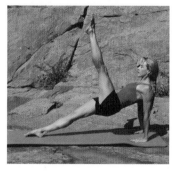

30. Leg Pull-Up, page 161

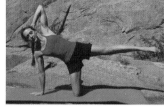

31. Kneeling Side Kicks, page 162

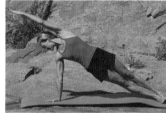

32. Side Bend, page 163

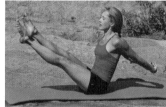

33. Boomerang, page 164

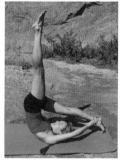

34. Control Balance, page 167

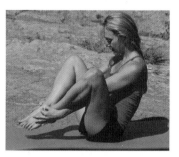

35. Seal, page 166

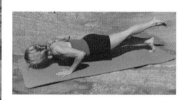

36. One-Leg Push-Ups, page 170

Dumbbells Routine— Upper-Body and Abdominal Muscles

This places an emphasis on upper-body and core conditioning. Allow 15 to 20 minutes to complete.

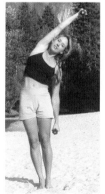

1. Side-to-Side, page 205

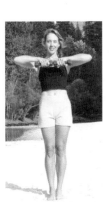

2.
Zip-Ups,
page 210

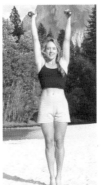

6.
Arm
Circles,
page 194

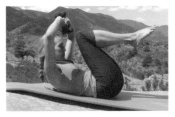

10. Elementary Backstroke,
page 186

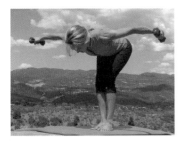

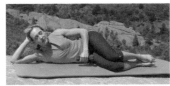

7. Rotator Cuff, page 201

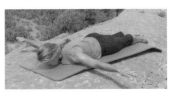

11. Coordination, page 182

3. Bug, page 195

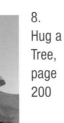

8.
Hug a
Tree,
page
200

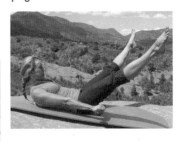

12. T-Bird, page 192

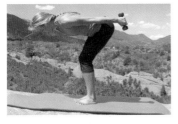

4. Triceps Kickbacks,
page 208

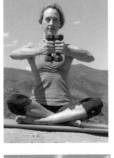

13.
Wrist
Curls,
page
209

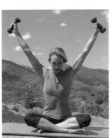

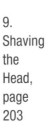

9.
Shaving
the
Head,
page
203

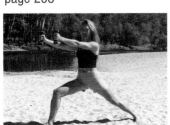

5. Side Lunges, page 179

For athletes, injuries are common. Aggravating an existing injury can slow progress and cause other problems. Tight muscles, such as hamstrings and shoulders, may require modifications as well. Below are some suggestions for modifying exercises. If none of the mentioned modifications do the trick, seek the advice of a qualified Pilates instructor or omit the exercise altogether.

Back Injuries: Seek the advice of your physician before beginning your routine. Depending upon your injury, some types of spinal movements such as flexion, extension, rotation, or side bending may be off-limits.

Neck Injury: If lifting your head while doing abdominal exercises causes tension or pain, rest it on the mat and consider placing a small pillow under your head. Remember, keep your neck and head in proper alignment to your spine.

Shoulder Injuries: Avoid adding resistance or putting weight on your arms and shoulders if it causes pain. Also, avoid bringing your arms overhead or in other positions that cause pain. Instead, modify an exercise by bringing your arms into a pain-free zone.

Wrist Injury: Avoid putting pressure on your wrists. If an exercise requires being on your wrists, prop yourself up on your elbows. In the case of push-ups, consider making your hands into fists and keeping a straight wrist.

Tight Hamstrings: When attempting to sit up with your legs out straight, if your back rounds, sit on a cushion, phone book, or rolled-up mat. It's more important to keep a straight spine than to sit on the floor with your legs at a 90-degree angle.

Weak Core: To create additional back support while doing exercises such as the Hundred, bend your knees and bring your legs closer to your body. As a general rule, the farther your legs are from your body, the more core strength is required to support your lower back. Never allow your lower back to arch off the floor while doing a Pilates exercise.

Glossary

Pilates and Basic Anatomy Terminology

Abdominals: Four muscles, transverses abdominus, internal obliques, external obliques, and the rectus abdominus, that provide support for the spine and stabilize the torso for movement.

Agonist: The primary muscle(s) that are used to create a movement.

Anchoring: Pilates cue that describes the action of creating oppositional energy. For example, reaching down through your feet while simultaneously reaching with your arms creates an anchor similar to the hand that holds a kite or the anchor of a boat. Anchoring helps to create length in the spine and decompression in the joints.

Antagonist: Muscles opposite to the ones required to execute a movement. These muscles lengthen to allow movement of the bones.

Anterior: The front side of the body.

Biceps: Four muscles, biceps brachii, brachialis, brachioradialis, and pronator teres, that flex the arm at the elbow joint and facilitate flexion of the elbow and shoulder joints.

Bones: Provide the framework for the body and act as levers for movement.

Cadence: Revolutions per minute for a running stride, pedaling stroke, or swimming stroke.

Calves: Two muscles on the back side of the lower leg: gastronemius and the soleus. These muscles stabilize the ankles.

Cartilage: Connective tissue that provides cushion between two bones.

C-Curl: Pilates cue for exercises such as the Hundred and One-Leg Stretch. To C-curl, begin by lying on your back, lifting your head to look toward your feet, and curl up to the base of your shoulder blades. Your gaze should be forward with a small space between your chin and chest.

Center of Gravity: The place where we find our center of balance in the body. Center of gravity is located at the pelvis in front of the sacrum at approximately half of our height.

Central Axis: An imaginary vertical line that runs through the center of the body creating a reference for alignment of your head, shoulders, and pelvis.

Cervical Spine: The seven vertebrae that make up the neck.

Deltoids: Three triangular-shaped muscles that lie at the top of the upper arm.

Dorsal Flexion: Movement of the foot that brings the toes closer to the knees. Requires activating the muscles of the shins while stretching the muscles of the calves.

Erector Spinae: Small muscles that run the length of your spine facilitating extension of the spine. Utilized in maintaining proper posture as well as to back bend.

Eversion: The action of the foot when the outer border lifts. If you were standing, this would mean lifting the outside edges of your feet off the floor.

Extension: Movement that increases the angle between the bones or other body parts. Back bending is an example of extension.

Extensors: Muscles engaged in creating extension movement. Back muscles and triceps are examples of extensors.

Flexion: Movement that decreases the angle between the bones or other body parts. An example of flexion would be to round your spine or flex your biceps.

Flexors: Muscles that assist in flexion of the joints or spine. Abdominals and biceps are considered flexors.

Hamstrings: Three muscles on the back of the upper leg, biceps femoris, semitendinosus, and semimembranosus, that bend the knee joint and assist in rotating the lower leg and in extending the femoral joint.

Hip Abductors: Consist of the following muscles: gluteus medius, minimus, and maximus, tensor fasciae latae, piriformis, obturators, gemilli, and sartorius. The hip abductors move the legs away from the midline of the body and assist in stabilizing the leg and aligning the knee and hip joints.

Hip Adductors: Consist of the following muscles: adductor magnus, adductor longus, adductor brevis, pectineus, gracilis, psoas, and iliacus. The hip adductors move the legs across the midline of the body. Inner thigh muscles function to stabilize the leg and align the knee and hip joints.

Hip Extensors: Include the gluteus medius, minimus, and maximus. Creates extension of the leg at the hip joint.

Hip Flexors: Consist of two muscles: the iliacus and the psoas major; together they are known as the iliopsoas. They engage to lift the leg upward. Tightness in the hip flexors can create lower-back tightness.

Hollowing Out: Pilates cue that describes the act of pulling the abdominal muscles in and upward to form a visible hollow in the belly.

Iliotibial Band: A band of strong fibrous tissue that runs from your hip along the outside of your leg. The gluteal muscles and the tensor fascia lata muscle attach to the top of this tissue.

Inversion: The action of tilting your foot so the inner border lifts. If you were standing, this would mean rolling onto the outside edges of your feet.

Joints: The place where two bones meet.

Knitting Together: A Pilates cue that refers to drawing the front of your ribs together. This helps prevent the lower back from arching.

Lateral: The outside border of a limb or part that is farthest from the midline of the body.

Lateral Flexion: Also known as side bending of the spine.

Latissimus Dorsi (Lats): Connects the upper part of the arm to the spinal column. It is used any time the body is lifted upward by the arms or when the arms push downward. When overly tight, they can compromise the integrity of the shoulder by causing the head of the humerus to rotate too far forward in its socket.

Ligaments: Attach bones to bones and function to stabilize joints.

Lordosis: Also known as swayback. Lordosis is characterized by an exaggerated curve of the lumbar spine.

Lumbar Spine: Refers to the lower five vertebrae of the spine.

Medial: The inside border of a limb or the part that is closest to your midline.

Navel to Spine: Pilates cue used to engage your deepest layer of core musculature: the transverses abdominus.

Neutral Pelvis: Refers to a position of the pelvis in relationship to the spine that adds support and stability.

Obliques: Abdominal muscles that facilitate rotation, side bending, and flexion.

Pectorals: Consist of two muscles: pectoralis major and minor. Both are important to the stability of the shoulder.

Peroneals: Muscles along the outside of the lower leg that stabilize the leg at the foot as it hits the ground.

Pilates V: Pilates cue that refers to the position of the feet in a "V" shape while standing so the heels are together and the feet are turned out. To properly create the Pilates V requires external rotation of the leg from the hip and drawing the backs of the legs together.

Plantar Flexion: Pointing the toes. Plantar flexion activates the muscles of the calves and lengthens the muscles of the shins.

Plumb Line: Pilates cue for creating proper alignment. Refers to an imaginary line drawn through the center of the body from the ears to the ankles.

Posterior: Refers to the back side of the body.

Powerhouse: A term coined by Joseph Pilates that refers to the muscles of the abdomen, hips, and lower back.

Q-Angle: The angle from the front side of your hip bone to the center of your kneecap and from the center of your kneecap to just below it, where the patellar tendon inserts.

Quadriceps: Powerful group of muscles on the front upper thigh that straighten the leg while striding. Strong quadriceps help maintain proper tracking of the hips, knees, and ankles.

Rhomboids: Two muscles that attach your shoulder blades to your spine. They retract and assist in rotating your blades downward.

Rotator Cuff: Consists of four muscles: supraspinatus, infraspinatus, terres minor, and subscapularis. The rotator cuff functions to stabilize the head of the humerus in the shoulder socket.

Sacrum: Five fused vertebrae at the base of the spine that form a flat, wedge-shaped bone above the tailbone.

Scapula: Also known as the shoulder blade, the scapulae are two triangular-shaped bones forming the back of the shoulder girdle.

Scooping: Pilates cue that refers to hollowing out the belly by drawing the abdominal muscles inward and upward under the rib cage.

Serratus Anterior: Runs along the outside of the rib cage below your armpit. When reaching overhead, it rotates your shoulder blades upward and provides strength to the upper back and shoulders.

Spinal Articulation: The ability to differentiate and articulate the vertebrae of your spine.

Spinal Extensors: Muscles that extend the spine in movements such as back bending.

Spinal Imprinting: Joseph Pilates' protégé Eve Gentry is credited for the concept of spinal imprinting. Spinal imprinting means to feel and distinguish as many vertebrae of your spine as possible as you roll down onto a mat. It is useful for improving alignment, awareness, and creating decompression in the spine. This concept applies to all rolling exercises.

Sternum: Also known as the breastbone. The place where the ribs connect into the front of the body.

Tendons: Connect muscles to bones.

Thoracic Spine: Refers to the middle 12 vertebrae of the spine. It is also the place where the ribs connect into the back side of the body.

Tracking: Refers to the alignment of your joints in relationship to other joints, such as the ankles, kneecaps, and hips, while engaging in an activity such as walking or riding a bike.

Trapezius: Large triangular back muscle that connects into the base of the head, the shoulder girdle, and down at the twelfth thoracic vertebra. It is so large that muscular work is referred to as originating from the upper, mid-, and lower trapezius.

Triceps: A large three-headed muscle on the back side of the upper arm, making up approximately 60 percent of the upper arm's mass. The triceps are engaged when straightening the arm. Maintaining their strength helps to maintain the integrity of the elbow and prevent lateral epicondylitis.

Vastus Medialus Oblique (VMO): The inner portion of the quadriceps helps to maintain proper tracking of the kneecap. Adequate VMO strength can often mitigate knee injuries such as Patellofemoral Pain Syndrome (Runner's Knee) and Chondromalacia Patella.

Winging: Shoulder blades that protrude from the back. Winging is caused by lack of muscle balance in the shoulder muscles.

Wrapping: Pilates cue for engaging the outer hip and inner thigh muscles while the legs are turned out or in a Pilates V.

Wrist Extensors: Muscles that run along the top side of the forearm. They assist in bringing the back of the hand closer to the forearm.

Wrist Flexors: Muscles that run along the bottom side of the forearm. They assist in making a fist.

Zipping Up: Pilates cue that is sometimes used to engage either the abdominals or the backs of the thighs. To engage the abdominals, pretend you are putting on a tight pair of jeans fresh out of the dryer and draw your abdominal muscles upward and inward. Joseph Pilates' protégé Kathy Grant is credited for this terrific cue. To engage the backs of the legs, pretend as though you had a zipper running down your legs and zip it up.

References and Recommended Reading

Al Juang, Chungliang and Jerry Lynch. *Thinking Body, Dancing Mind.* New York: Bantam Books, 1992.

Burke, Edmund R. and Ed Pavelka. *The Complete Book of Long-Distance Cycling.* Emmaus, PA: Rodale, 2000.

Calais-Germain, Blandine. *Anatomy of Movement.* Seattle: Eastland Press, 1993.

Carlson, Julia. *A Woman's Guide to Snowboarding.* Camden, ME: Ragged Mountain Press, 1999.

Covey, Stephen. *The Seven Habits of Highly Effective People.* New York: Simon and Schuster, 1989.

Elling, Mark R. *The All-Mountain Skier.* Camden, ME: Ragged Mountain Press, 2003.

Ellis, Joe. *Running Injury-Free.* Emmaus, PA: Rodale, 1994.

Frediani, Paul and Harold Harb. *Ski Flex.* Long Island City, NY: Hatherleigh Press, 2003.

Friel, Joe. *The Triathlete's Training Bible.* Boulder, CO: VeloPress, 2004.

Guten, Gary N. *Injuries in Outdoor Recreation.* Guilford, CT: Falcon, 2005.

Hörst, Eric J. *Training for Climbing.* Guilford, CT: Globe Pequot Press, 2003.

Jackson, Eric. *Whitewater Paddling.* Mechanicsburg, PA: Stackpole Books, 1999.

Levy, Allan M. *Sports Injury Handbook.* Hoboken, NJ: John Wiley and Sons, Inc., 1993.

Musnick, David and Mark Pierce. *Conditioning for Outdoor Fitness.* Seattle: The Mountaineers, 1999.

Parker, Paul. *Free-Heel Skiing.* Seattle: The Mountaineers Books, 2002.

Pilates, Joseph. *Pilates' Return to Life through Contrology,* 1945.

Prater, Gene. *Snowshoeing: From Novice to Master.* Seattle: The Mountaineers, 2002.

Robbins, Anthony. *Awaken the Giant Within.* New York: Fireside, 1991.

Sagar, Heather Reynolds. *Climbing Your Best.* Mechanicsburg, PA: Stackpole Books, 2001.

Schmidt, Richard A. and Craig A. Wrisberg. *Motor Learning and Performance.* Champaign, IL: Human Kinetics, 2000.

Sweigard, Lulu E. *Human Movement Potential.* Lanham, MD: University Press of America, 1974.

Tarpinian, Steve. *The Triathlete's Guide to Swim Training.* Boulder, CO: VeloPress, 2005.

Wallenfels, Lynda. *The Triathlete's Guide to Bike Training.* Boulder, CO: VeloPress, 2004.

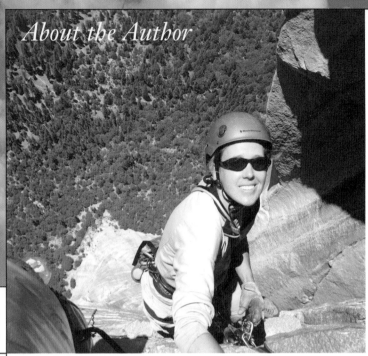

About the Author

Lauri Ann Stricker graduated from the University of Denver with a master's degree in business administration. After spending many years helping small businesses succeed, Lauri discovered Pilates and since then has worked passionately to help individuals create better fitness programs. Lauri has worked extensively with outdoor athletes helping them to avoid injury and to reach peak levels of performance. Lauri is the founder of Blue Sky Pilates and Evergreen Pilates. When she is not teaching and writing, she enjoys spending time beneath the great blue sky pursuing athletic adventures.